Linda Abbott

THE HULL HOME FIRE

LINDA ABBOTT

THE HULL HOME FIRE

FLANKER PRESS LIMITED

ST. JOHN'S

Library and Archives Canada Cataloguing in Publication

Abbott, Linda, 1951-, author
The Hull Home fire / Linda Abbott.

Issued in print and electronic formats.
ISBN 978-1-77117-262-2 (pbk.).--ISBN 978-1-77117-263-9 (epub).--
ISBN 978-1-77117-264-6 (kindle).--ISBN 978-1-77117-265-3 (pdf)

1. Hull Nursing Home--Fire, 1948. 2. Nursing homes--Fires and fire prevention--Newfoundland and Labrador--St. John's--History--20th century. 3. Fires--Casualties--Newfoundland and Labrador--St. John's--Biography. I. Title.

TH9445.A4A23 2013 363.3709718'1 C2013-905571-1
C2013-905572-X

PRINTED IN CANADA

Cover Design: Graham Blair Edited by Paul Butler

Flanker Press Ltd.
PO Box 2522, Station C
St. John's, NL
Canada

TELEPHONE: (709) 739-4477 FAX: (709) 739-4420 TOLL-FREE: 1-866-739-4420
WWW.FLANKERPRESS.COM

9 8 7 6 5 4 3 2 1

Canada Canada Council for the Arts Conseil des Arts du Canada Newfoundland Labrador

We acknowledge the financial support of the Government of Canada through the Book Publishing Industry Development Program (BPIDP) for our publishing activities; the Canada Council for the Arts, which last year invested $157 million to bring the arts to Canadians throughout the country; the Government of Newfoundland and Labrador, Department of Tourism, Culture and Recreation.

For Uncle Joe, who always had a story to tell

For Aunt Betty, always ready with a joke

Chapter 1

HENRY GIBBS SAT DOWN AND sprinkled cinnamon over the steaming bowl of oatmeal. A slice and a half of toast made from his mother's freshly baked raisin bread lay on a side plate. "Mom, it's finally arrived." He shoved a piece of toast in his mouth as he took an envelope from his trousers pocket.

Alice Gibbs placed six strips of bacon in the frying pan one by one. The fat sizzled as she turned from the stove. "Good news, I take it," she said. Her smile revealed the slight gap in her top front teeth.

"What's that?" Tom Gibbs snapped from the doorway. His eyes bore into the envelope. Tom, an older version of his son, was tall and broad-shouldered. Years on the docks unloading cargo had left him trim and well-muscled. Almost fifty years old, his black hair showed no signs of grey. Green eyes, which sometimes sparkled with a smile, now chilled Henry. His arms were stiff at his side.

Henry's mouth went dry and he just managed to swallow the toast. He made to speak, but the words wouldn't come.

"Well?" Tom said, moving with long strides into the

kitchen. He pulled out a chair across from his son. The scraping throbbed in Henry's ears.

Alice picked up the faded blue teapot from the wood stove and hurried toward the table. "Tom, you're not yourself in the mornings until you've had a nice hot cup of tea."

"In a minute," Tom said, glaring at his son.

Henry's tongue stuck to his teeth as he drained the last of the tea from the saucer. "It . . . it's from a university in Canada," he said, meeting his father's icy stare.

"I told you to forget all that nonsense." Tom pounded his fist on the table. Henry's bowl of oatmeal danced near the edge.

"Goodness me!" Alice said. Startled, she jumped back a step, nearly losing her hold on the teapot. The cover rattled, then slipped off and crashed to the floor. Hot tea plopped over the rim, scalding her as it dripped down her hand. She cried out, dropping the pot back on the stove.

Tom sprang to his feet and took her injured hand gently in his. "I'm sorry, love," he said. "I didn't mean to frighten you." His face softened as he led his wife to the sink.

"This isn't like you, Tom," Alice said quietly, watching the cold water flow over the welts that covered all four fingers from the knuckles down.

Henry stared at the breakfast he normally finished off in minutes. His right knee tapped against the underside of the table.

Tom sighed. No one spoke as he reached for a jar of Vaseline from a shelf over the sink. He spread the yellowish gel over the blisters. "How's that?" he asked, keeping his head down.

Alice nodded. "Grand." She briefly caressed his cheek and waited for him to look at her. "It doesn't hurt anymore."

Tom gave a weak smile and picked up the teapot's cover, which had split down the centre. "I'll glue it back together," he said, laying it aside on the sink counter.

Alice returned to the stove and forked out the fried bacon one piece at a time with her uninjured hand. "Sit down," she said with an authoritative tone she rarely used. "It's best to discuss our son's news on a full stomach."

Tom took the chair he had vacated and fiddled with a knife. His eyes strayed to the envelope Henry gripped like it was a lifeline. The University of Toronto was printed in bold black letters in the top left corner. He ran a hand through his hair. "I told you not to apply."

Henry forced himself to look at his father. "I've been accepted."

Tom's eyelids fluttered.

Henry charged ahead. "For the medical department in the spring. Dad, I don't understand why you're so against me being a doctor."

"You're twenty-one, too old to bother about more book learning."

"It's much more than that."

"No! We can't afford it."

Henry's eyes brightened. "You won't have to spend a nickel, Dad. I've saved enough money for two semesters. I can get a part-time job to keep me going."

Tom's face darkened as he sat back into the chair and folded his arms across his thick chest. "What happens if you can't manage your studies and keep a job?" His voice was barely above a whisper.

"I'll make it work," Henry said. A pulse beat in his temple. "I can't give up the only chance I'll ever have to be a doctor."

Tom shook his head. “The docks weren’t good enough for you? Well, my boy, it’s put a roof over our heads and food on the table.”

“Dad, it’s not that.” Henry glanced at his mother for support. His heart dropped at the sad expression on her face just before she turned away. His eyes spun back to his father. “Being a doctor means everything to me. As soon as I’m certified I’ll come home to start my practice.”

Tom laughed—a sound that expressed neither joy nor comfort. “I’ve heard that before,” he mumbled. His gaze drifted somewhere over Henry’s head.

Here it comes, Henry thought. The story he’d heard since he was a child. The story he dreaded to hear yet again.

“My brother sat at a kitchen table and babbled the same drivel as you.” He blinked and leaned toward his son. “So my parents saved every penny to send him to medical school even though my mother wasn’t too keen on the idea. He left and never returned. Just a letter every now and then. It broke my mother’s heart and my father died of a stroke from working two jobs. Mike didn’t even come home for either of their funerals.” His breathing was laboured. “I prayed you’d never turn out like my ungrateful older brother.”

“Dad, please listen to me.”

Tom shut his eyes and the fine lines at the corners deepened. “I don’t care what you do,” he said. Without looking at Henry he stood up and walked out of the kitchen. The back door opened and banged shut.

Alice sat down next to her son and glanced out the window into the yard. Tom rammed a fist into a row of icicles as he strode past. Three cracked off and fell to the ground.

“Dad’s really mad this time.”

"Your father's not thinking straight." Alice turned to her son. "He never wanted you to waste your life on the docks."

"I know."

"He doesn't mean to be so hard on you, either."

Henry pushed the bowl of cold oatmeal away. "You'd think he'd be proud I want to be a doctor."

"Tom idolized his only brother." Alice sighed, a long-drawn-out breath. "We were married a whole year before he told me about Mike."

"I'm not Uncle Mike," Henry said. "I'd never abandon my family."

"Tom was hurt. You're well aware what a stubborn old coot he can sometimes be. He tore up all Mike's letters without reading a single one after his mother's death."

"But—"

"You're our only child," Alice said, interrupting Henry. "He's afraid he'll never see you again." She squeezed his hand. "Give him time to get used to the idea."

"Mom, he's been angry with his brother over forty years. He'll never get used to the idea." Henry's jaw tightened. "I won't throw away this one chance."

Alice gently rubbed his shoulder. "You shouldn't. I'll do my best to make him see reason." She looked out the window once more. Tom gathered wood for the stove, slapping the chopped pieces into the crook of his arm. He hadn't taken the time to put on a coat. "Finish your breakfast before your father comes in. We'll talk later."

Henry hurried along the sidewalk. At six foot three, his second-hand winter coat, the style worn to mid-calf, barely reached to his knees. The grey woollen cap pulled down over his ears wasn't much comfort against the wind snapping his turned-up collar against his red, numbed cheeks. The air stung his eyes. He wiped away cold-induced tears before they turned to ice chips on his long dark lashes. With each step, his breath pooled into wispy clouds.

Henry shoved his hands into large pockets and ducked his head low as he stepped off the curb. He didn't bother to check for cars as there was never any traffic at six in the morning. He didn't hear the crunch of snow under his feet or notice the rows of red, green, and yellow attached houses jammed together like clumps of jujubes. The conversation—argument was a more accurate description—with his father played on his mind. The wind took his breath away as he turned onto Clifford Street, dragging his thoughts back to the present. His stomach growled with hunger. The sight of his father storming out of the kitchen had taken away his appetite. Henry could still see the look on his face. It was unbelievable that the most important decision of his life was his father's greatest disappointment. Cold air snaked down his neck. He shivered. If he didn't get inside soon, he was sure his nose would freeze and drop off. He squinted through half-closed eyes at Walsh's Bakery a few steps away. The smell of baking bread intensified his hunger. He turned down Springdale Street and was never more thrilled to see Hull Home, his place of employment where he worked as an accountant. His fingers were so stiff he was hardly able to turn the doorknob.

Isaac Hull, a forty-year-old man of medium height with thinning brown hair, looked down the stairs. "It's only you," he said. A grey vest hugged his round stomach born of too much gravy and potatoes. He glanced at his watch. "I was expecting the delivery man from the bakery."

Henry hugged himself, rubbing the top of his arms as he

climbed to the second floor. "It must be the coldest winter on record," he said.

"That's what the radio says every time I turn it on."

"You're here early, Mr. Hull," Henry said. He hung his coat on a hall hook outside the large office and went inside with his boss.

"I stayed overnight. The godforsaken stove's acting up again." Isaac pulled out his watch again. "There's a heap of hungry people waiting for breakfast. I need seven loaves of bread right away."

"At least there'll be hot toast," Henry said. "Even if there's no tea to wash it down."

Mr. Hull narrowed his eyes at Henry. "We make do in an emergency." A *rat-tat-tat* sounded on the front door. "That better be the bakery. I called more than an hour ago," he said and hurried to the front entrance as a louder thump filled the Home. A frigid blast of wind washed over him when he pulled open the door.

"Morning, Mr. Hull." It was Fred Russell, the bakery delivery man, his smile wide.

"About time," Isaac said and almost threw the money at the man.

"I left as soon as the bread popped out of the ovens." Fred passed over the loaves wrapped in brown paper tied with white string. "They're still piping hot. We received an extra big order from Hotel Newfoundland. A group of government officials are up from Canada to haggle over Confederation."

Isaac grunted a reply and went up the stairs leaving Fred staring after him.

Henry darted out from the office. "The stove's on the blink again," he said. "It's put Mr. Hull in a right crooked mood."

"You don't say," Fred said, wiping his feet on the mat. "The residents must be good and fed up with nothing but toast most mornings."

"I haven't heard any complaints," Henry said.

Fred took a plump paper bag from an inside pocket and mounted the stairs. "Here's some crinkle scraps for you." The cake-like yellow dessert was Henry's favourite.

"Thanks ever so much," Henry said, reminded once again how hungry he was.

"Always a pleasure, my boy."

Henry returned to the office and munched on a crinkle while he worked on the books. He ate three before the hunger pangs subsided.

A sudden draft signalled someone had entered the building. Henry looked up to see Mary Norris. She worked from six in the morning to seven at night as a cleaner and all-around handywoman. "Morning, Henry," she said. The twenty-year-old crossed the hall to the office and stood in the doorway. "You're up with the birds."

Henry noticed the dark circles under her eyes. He stood up from the desk and ran a thumb under each one. "You look like you haven't slept in days. What happened?"

"The stove leaked oil again last night just as I was about to leave. We had to put a bucket under the valve to catch the drippings." She made a face and held out red, dry hands. "It took me an hour to scrub the canvas and get rid of the stink."

Henry indicated the kitchen with a turn of his eyes and put a finger to his lips. "Mr. Hull spent the night here," he mouthed.

"That's becoming a regular thing," Mary mouthed back.

Henry returned to the topic at hand, his voice low. "For a new stove it's been nothing but trouble."

“A few weeks after it was bought, the valves had to be replaced,” Mary whispered. “Which is odd.” She sneaked a look down the hall to the kitchen. “Valves are the one thing that last quite a while on a stove.”

“Good thing your grandfather was a trained mechanic and taught you everything he knows.”

“Anytime I mention the stove Mr. Hull tells me it’s taken care of and to get on with my work.” Mary chewed her bottom lip. “Did you hear back from the university?”

“Yes,” Henry said after a slight hesitation. “I was going to tell you tonight.”

Mary’s eyes seemed to sink into her face. “What did your father say?” she asked quietly.

“He’s fit to be tied.”

Henry reached for her hands, but she pulled away. His heart flip-flopped. “You know I’ll do almost anything to be a doctor.”

“You’ll need more money than you have saved up,” Mary said. Her voice sounded artificial. Tiny beads of sweat bubbled on her forehead. She opened her coat and yanked off her wool hat. Straight blonde hair tumbled to her shoulders. “Mr. Hull won’t stand for me chatting it up with you all day.”

Henry saw what looked like a silver chain partially concealed by her sweater. “What’s that?”

Mary pulled the chain all the way out and fingered a silver half-moon. “Gramps gave it to me.” She turned her head to the side and her face became hidden in a shadow. “Two days before his massive heart attack.”

“Oh,” Henry said. “I didn’t mean to upset you.” He cleared his throat. “Why didn’t you show it to me?”

Mary met his gaze. “I guess it slipped my mind.” She tucked

the chain inside her sweater. "Gramps wouldn't want me to mope around on his account."

TOM CAME IN FROM THE yard with an armload of chopped wood. His lips were blue, and his teeth chattered like a woodpecker hard at work. Moisture dangled like a teardrop from the tip of his reddened nose.

"Feel better?" Alice said. She leaned back against the counter and crossed one ankle over the other. "A grown man storming out into the freezing cold without a coat because he didn't like what he heard."

Tom dumped the wood into the bin next to the stove. "I don't want to talk about Henry right now." His hand shook as he took a handkerchief out of his pocket and blew his nose.

Alice put a bowl of porridge on the table. "Sit down. You have to get hot food inside you." She took her coat from the back of the chair. "It'll serve you right if you end up with pneumonia."

Tom glanced up at her. "Off to see your mother at Hull Home?"

"Of course."

"Why she'd rather live with sick people is beyond me. She should be here with her own folk."

"Tom, how many times do I have to tell you that Hull Home is a boarding house as well as a nursing home?" She unhooked her purse from around the doorknob. "Mom doesn't want to be a burden to us. Besides, she has friends there she's known for most of her life."

Tom dug into the porridge. "The Department of Public Health has no right to allow TB cases to live with healthy old folk. That doesn't sound proper to me."

"I think it's a grand place," Alice said. "They even look after the darling children of unwed mothers until they are adopted."

"Come on, love. They want the extra money, you mean. The Salvation Army does that for free. I bet Mr. Hull bent Henry's ear about this doctor business in the hope he'll volunteer there."

"Young Mary Norris says he really cares about the residents."

"She has no other choice but to say that, because she's the only one bringing in money since her grandfather passed." Tom slapped jam on cold toast. "Our son has shown beyond a doubt how much she means to him, with this doctor business."

Alice tweaked her husband's chin. "Not many men want their mother-in-law underfoot."

"Don't forget your scarf." Tom plucked it from the floor, wrapped it around her neck, and planted a quick peck on her forehead.

Alice smiled. "Won't be long, love."

"Say hello to your mother for me," Tom called as she stepped outside and set off for Hull Home. Six days a week she made the ten-minute walk to visit her mother. Dorothy Gatherall—or Dot, as she preferred—spent every Sunday with her daughter's family. Alice ran across the street. The cold air scratched her throat. Despite two pairs of gloves her fingers tingled. She rushed around the corner and collided with a man. He was fifty years old and below average height, with thick brown, greying hair.

"Mrs. Gibbs," Fred Russell said, holding out his arms to steady her. He chuckled. "Sorry I bumped into you."

Alice shuffled from foot to foot on the rock-hard snow. "I'm on the way to visit my mother."

"A word to the wise," Fred said. "The stove's giving trouble again."

Alice rolled her eyes. “I take it Mr. Hull’s in a foul mood.”

“You could say that.”

“Do me a favour, Fred. If you see Tom, don’t tell him. This’ll give him more ammunition to badmouth the Home.”

Chapter 2

"WHY ARE YOU LATE?" ISAAC griped. He knelt on the floor, his head and shoulders concealed behind the stove.

"I'm sorry," Mary said. "My migraine was so bad it kept me awake most of the night." She shed her sweater and hung it on the back of a chair. "I'll make the toast right away."

Isaac rose slowly to his feet and brushed dust off his knees. "Get on with it, then. The building inspector and the fire superintendent will be here at eight. I want everyone fed by then."

Mary untied the string around the bread and threw the brown paper in the garbage next to the sink. Isaac strutted down the hall to the office. "The stove would have to give out today," he grumbled. "Where's the bloody mechanic?"

Dot Gatherall strolled into the kitchen. "Our distinguished leader is in fine form this morning," she said as she took a butter knife out of the drawer. "Let me give you a hand, dearie."

Mary adjusted her apron more securely around her waist. "Mr. Hull will be right mad at me if I let a resident help fix breakfast. You saw how crooked he was this morning."

"Nonsense," Dot said, taking a slab of butter out of the fridge. "You shouldn't be expected to prepare breakfast for over fifty people all by yourself. Why isn't Mr. Hull helping out?"

Mary frowned. "The stove's giving trouble and he's worried about the inspection."

"Well," Dot said. "That's even more reason he should be in here with you." She patted Mary's arm. "Never you mind. We'll do just fine on our own."

A loud knock sounded on the front door. "Please let that be the mechanic," Mary said, darting down the stairs. She returned with Gordon Freeman, a stove mechanic who worked with Monroe Machinery and Equipment Company.

Dot smiled at the young man. "Good to see you again so soon, Gordon."

He placed his tool bag on the floor by the stove. "I'm called in so often to repair the stove my missus says I should move in," he said with a straight face.

Dot wiggled her eyebrows at him. "There's an extra bed in my room." She found a tray in the cupboard over the fridge for the batch of toast and carried it to the dining room. Mary poked more bread in the two-door toaster.

"Let's see what the trouble is this time," Gordon said, pulling tools out of his bag. "Looks like someone's been tampering with the carburetor." He turned to Mary. "Come take a look."

Mary crouched down next to the mechanic and examined the trip valve he indicated. "It's been tied down to keep it open," she said.

"Which, as you are well aware, Mary, means more oil is flowing than should be." He pointed to a fuel supply pipe. "That's leaking." A small puddle of oil had formed on the floor.

Mary sat back on her heels. “I saw Mr. Hull tinkering with the stove a little while ago.”

“How do you put up with him?” Gordon said. “He thinks he knows more than a real mechanic.”

“He doesn’t have a clue when it comes to mechanical things.”

“Mary!” Isaac growled, glaring down at her. “Get away from there. Hannah Smith needs her bedclothes changed immediately.”

“Yes, sir.” Mary jumped to her feet. “Poor Hannah sweats something awful when she has the flu.”

“Don’t be mad at Mary,” Gordon said as she scurried away. “I asked her to take a look.”

“She’s not your helper,” Isaac said. “She has enough work of her own to do.” He drummed his fingers on the table, watching Gordon’s every move. “That stove’s been nothing but a bother since the day I purchased it. Needs more looking after than a newborn.” Isaac hauled out his pocket watch. “Are you done?”

Gordon tightened a screw on the trip valve. “For now.”

Isaac’s eyes narrowed into slits. “Maybe it’s time you learned how to fix the damn stove once and for all.”

“Mr. Hull, you’ve got to stop tinkering with the carburetor. Oil’s leaking to the floor because of it.” The mechanic cleaned the greasy mess from his hands. “Flames will get outside the stove through the water pipes if you don’t. Too much oil causes high temperatures and extra gases.”

“Thank you, thank you,” Isaac said. “Now, if you don’t mind, see yourself out. I have important business to attend to.”

“Of course,” Gordon said to Mr. Hull’s retreating back. “Don’t I always?”

Dot brought the empty tray back to the kitchen. “Gordon,

I . . ." She paused and looked at him as if unsure of what to say. "I heard what you said to Mr. Hull about the stove. It sounded awful dangerous to me."

Gordon collected his tools from the floor. "It is, Mrs. Gatherall. I sure hope he heeds my warning this time."

Mary descended the stairs as the mechanic opened the front door to leave. "Have a good day, Gordon."

"Keep an eye on the stove, Mary," he said as the door closed behind him, and left with the tool bag tucked under an arm. Two men approached the home. Gordon tipped his hat to them. "Morning, gents."

Fire Superintendent Fred Vivian, the tallest of the pair, rang the doorbell. Mr. Hull scooted out of his office, his wife close at hand. "Come in. Come in, gentlemen," he said, a broad smile plastered across his face. Mary returned to the kitchen and busied herself with making more toast.

City Building Inspector Cahill pulled off his scarf.

"It's best to leave that on," Isaac said. "We have to go outside to get to the Annex."

"Well now," Cahill said, "that's not very convenient, is it? Especially during the winter. By the way, are you the owners of the building?"

"No. We pay the Noah family sixty-five dollars a month for rent. Mr. Wylie, a commercial agent, occupies the first floor. His furnace heats the whole building."

Mrs. Hull stuck out her chin. "We pay him three hundred dollars a year," she added. "A very generous amount if you ask me."

Superintendent Vivian sniffed several times. "You've painted recently," he said, looking over the walls. "The smell is still quite potent."

"My God, man. That has to be removed immediately." He looked at Mrs. Hull, her face devoid of any humour. "Has any poor old soul stumbled over that stove yet?"

"Indeed not. Safety is one of our main priorities."

They started up the stairs, Cahill in the lead. "There's hardly enough room for one person at a time," he said. "My shoulders are scant inches from the walls."

Vivian wrote down a few more words. "An exceptionally narrow space for sure," he said.

"Which meets the required three-feet width," Mrs. Hull said and walked the group down the hall. "Gentlemen, I'm confident that you'll agree the rooms are clean and the residents well attended to." Vivian and Cahill filled out page after page as they scrutinized each room. Mary travelled from room to room, hanging up clothes and sweeping floors, her ears alert in an attempt to hear the conversation between the Hulls and the Fire Department officials.

A raspy cough scraped into the air. "That's Mrs. Duggan," Isaac said. "She's recovering nicely from tuberculosis."

Mary rushed into her room and poured water from the jug on the bedside table. "This'll help," she said, holding the glass to Mrs. Duggan's mouth.

"Thank you, my dear," the old lady croaked.

Mr. Hull smiled. "As you have observed, we have a very sympathetic staff."

"How many such cases do you have?" Cahill said.

"Eighteen."

Mrs. Hull clasped her hands together. "All doing grand," she said.

Cahill scribbled down another line. "I haven't seen a nurse on our rounds," he said. "Where are they?"

Mr. Hull went back into the hall. "The night nurse went home sick. The other two are due at nine."

They proceeded to the far room on the right. Isaac extracted a key from his pocket.

"Why's the door locked?" Vivian asked.

Mrs. Hull smiled, a mere rise of thin lips. "Old Mr. Newhook wanders about. We don't want him falling down the stairs."

"My Lord," Vivian said, looking at Isaac. "It's never a smart idea to lock residents in their rooms. In case of fire." He scanned the room from the hallway. "There are seven occupants in there. I've seen bigger closets."

"You're right," Cahill said. "The room would be overcrowded with three people."

"Take a closer look," Mrs. Hull said. "There's ample room."

"I disagree, madam."

"Mr. Cahill, I'll have you know our residents are happy folk who frequently visit each other's rooms."

Superintendent Vivian closed his notepad. "Mr. and Mrs. Hull. Thank you for your time and co-operation. We'll write up an official report with our recommendations."

HENRY STRETCHED AND LAY DOWN his pencil. He knew it had to be five o'clock by the rumbles in his stomach. "Mr. Hull, your wife will come looking for you if you stay late again."

"Not in this godforsaken weather she won't."

"See you in the morning," Henry said, and heard a desk drawer squeak open as he left the office. He shot a glance over his shoulder in time to see Isaac take out a bottle of screech. Henry grinned to himself and walked outside to a sky twinkling here and there with a few stars. A grey and white husky, hobbling alongside his ninety-year-old master, stopped and stared up at Henry. The animal's crystal blue eyes hadn't dimmed with age. "Good evening to you, Mr. Duggan," Henry said.

The old man measured five foot five and weighed a little over a hundred pounds. Fragile in appearance, he was fitter than a man thirty years his junior. A dark green wool cap covered a full head of wavy silver hair. The only visible wrinkles on his face formed at the corners of his mouth when he smiled.

"Hello, young man."

Henry rubbed the dog behind its ear. "How's your arthritis, Rusty boy?"

Mr. Duggan looked down at his friend and pet. "As good as can be expected for an ancient codger like him." Rusty licked his wrist.

"It sure is cold," Henry said.

"Cold enough to take strips off your face."

"Gran told me that Mrs. Duggan's doing better."

"Eileen isn't coughing near so much and she's put on a pound or two." Ten years younger than her husband, she suffered from a recurring bout of tuberculosis. His voice grew soft. "Hull Home agrees with her more than the Sanatorium. She feels more like a guest than a patient."

"That's good," Henry said, clapping his gloved hands to keep warm. He marvelled how the cold didn't seem to affect the elderly gentleman.

Rusty barked and cantered to the Home's front door. Mr. Duggan tapped the side of his head with two fingers. "The master commands, I obey," he said, and hurried after the dog.

The icy air sliced into Henry's skin. The wind picked up.

"Henry."

He turned. The full moon highlighted Hull Home like a

spotlight. Mary Norris hurried toward him, massaging her temples. "You all right, Mary?"

"I have another migraine." She scrunched up her forehead. "Mr. Case took his sweet time to paint the place. The second I get a whiff of the fumes my head begins to pound." Mary clutched her stomach. "I feel like throwing up, too."

"The smell is awful bad. Maybe you should go home."

"I don't work, I don't get paid. Anyway, Mr. Hull asked me to call you back."

"Mary, I want to talk to you about medical . . ." Henry's voice trailed away as she turned and walked back up the street to the Home. He remained rooted to the spot until the chill drove him into movement. The office empty, he ambled to the kitchen at the end of the hall. She was filling the kettle with water. "Mary, have you seen Mr. Hull?"

Curtly, she answered, "I'm not his keeper."

Henry blinked. "Sorry."

Mary turned from the stove. "He's probably with one of the residents." Her voice softened a fraction. "I was just about to make a cup of tea for myself." She brought down a package of tea leaves from the cupboard. "I hope the stove lasts long enough to get supper under way."

"Maybe it's high time Mr. Hull replaced it."

Mary groaned, her eyes on the dishcloths lining the pipes behind the stove. "I keep taking those off. Mr. Hull insists on putting them back."

"Mom never does that," Henry said. "She's afraid they might catch fire."

Mary whipped away the row of dry dishcloths and tidied them into a drawer. "There was some lot wrong with the stove," she said, and explained the details.

"Mr. Hull's aware how dangerous all that is. Right?"

"You'd be some idiot if you didn't." Mary sat down and folded her hands on the table, a faraway look on her face.

Henry stared at her full lips, slightly apart. His eyes travelled to the pug nose splattered with the occasional freckle. Such a pretty nose, he thought, and he wondered why he had teased her about it when they were youngsters. Steam pumped from the kettle spout, breaking Henry's trance. "You know I applied to medical school," he said. "So let's talk about it."

"Later. Right now I have a more immediate concern on my mind." Mary sighed long and deep. "Have you forgotten about the big inspection today? It didn't seem like they were too pleased with any of the conditions here." She tutted. "Mrs. Hull acted offended at their concerns."

"That's no surprise."

"Who'll feed my mother and Dougie if I lose my job?" Mary held her head high. "I don't want my little brother to have to quit school and work for scraps."

"I know it's been tough since your father left," Henry said, then paused. "Now your grandfather's gone as well."

Mary flashed dark eyes at him. "Don't ever speak of Gramps in the same sentence with the bastard who walked out on his family."

Henry felt his face burn. "I'm sorry, Mary. I shouldn't have brought him up."

Her hands clenched into fists. "Dougie was only two years old when he took off. Damn right I don't want that excuse for a father mentioned in any connection with my grandfather."

Isaac appeared from nowhere. "Mary, didn't you already have a spell from work?"

She spun around on her chair, startled. "I needed strong tea to help this killer migraine."

"Well, get on with it, girl. I'll be back shortly to cook supper." He glanced at Henry. "Come along."

Invoices and bills were strewn over Henry's desk. "I didn't have time to go through them while you were off over Christmas," Isaac said. "I forgot to mention them to you earlier, and seeing as tomorrow is Saturday . . ."

Henry gawked at him. "Christmas? They should've been logged in and paid for last month."

"I pay you to work for me, young man," Isaac hiccupped. "Not to lecture me."

Henry pulled up the sleeves of his sweater and sorted through the stack to the sound of pots and pans clanging in the kitchen. Halfway through the pile, the smell of tomato soup wafted toward him. His head ached by the time he wrote down the last figure. He closed the accounts book and put it in the desk's top drawer.

"It's six-thirty," Mary said, standing over the desk, her arms full with clean bedclothes. "How's it going?"

Henry rubbed tired eyes with the heels of his hands. "That late! No wonder I'm starving enough to eat worms."

Mary smiled at their childhood expression and pulled a tea bun out of her apron pocket. "Chew on this to tide you over. Made them myself last night."

Henry looked toward the kitchen where Mr. Hull stirred a pot on the stove. "You'd think he'd hire a proper cook."

Mary shrugged. "Maybe he can't spare the money."

"Right," Henry said. "Just like the King of England can't afford a proper cook."

Mary giggled despite herself. "Don't let him hear you say that."

Henry reached up and brushed strands of hair away from her mouth. "Your laughter reminds me of Christmas bells."

Mary backed away. "I have work to do."

"I'll drop in on Gran before I go," Henry said, pretending not to notice the slight. He dashed downstairs to the side door and ran the short distance to the Annex, annoyed he had forgotten his coat. The wind blew him inside, displacing several of the small, framed pictures strung along both walls. He manoeuvred around the stove and climbed the stairs two at a time.

"Gran," Henry called when he reached the room she shared with three women. Two of the three doors were blocked with sideboards. Night tables and armchairs cramped the already crowded space.

"She not's here," a voice called from across the hall.

Henry recognized Eileen Duggan's soft tone. The old lady held a raisin tea bun in one age-spotted hand and a cup of tea in the other. "Dot went out with your mother this morning." She took off wire-framed glasses and smiled at Henry. Her dark brown eyes seemed even darker against her pale skin.

"Thanks, Mrs. Duggan."

Eileen popped the last morsel of bun into her mouth. "That was delicious. Mary is a dear to bring in little treats for us."

Henry produced the one Mary had given him. "She's a good baker," he said, and devoured the bun. Heavy footsteps thumped in an irregular fashion toward the room. Dr. Kennedy slowed at the door.

"It's lovely to see you," Eileen said.

Henry nodded to the man from the Department of Health and Welfare. He was sent to the Home once a week to check on the patients. Sixty years old, tall, with slightly stooped shoulders, he limped to the bed. "I slipped on the darn ice getting out of my car. My hip will be bruised for a month."

"Gracious, Doctor," Eileen said. "Are you hurt bad?"

"Nothing too serious." He winked at Eileen. "How is my favourite patient today?"

A slight shade of pink crept up Eileen's face. "Grand, Doctor."

"Would you mind if Henry stayed while I examine you? Every bit of practice will come in handy for the boy."

"I don't mind at all. Dot's so proud of her grandson, the future doctor."

Dr. Kennedy warmed the stethoscope on the palm of his hand. He held it to Eileen's chest and explained the various sounds Henry should expect to hear. "Take a listen," he said, transferring the scope to her back.

Henry smiled. "Her lungs aren't congested as much."

The doctor poked a thermometer under Eileen's tongue. "Henry, have you told him yet?"

"He knows."

"And?"

Henry shook his head.

"He'll come 'round."

"I'd better get going," Henry said. "Mom will wonder where I am." He closed the bedroom door on the way out. At the bottom of the stairs he tripped on the stove and stumbled toward the door. He swore under his breath as Mary came in. "Damn stove should be moved to a safe place."

"It is a nuisance," Mary said. "But Mr. Hull won't hear tell of it being shifted anywhere else."

*

DOT GATHERALL SAT WITH TOM in his living room knitting a sweater for her only grandson. "Henry's late," she said, the needles clicking together.

Tom peered at her over the top of the *Evening Telegram*. He said nothing.

Dot put aside the knitting. "Think I'll see if Alice needs help with supper."

Tom closed the paper and lowered it to his lap. "Tell your daughter I know what you're both up to."

Dot put a finger on her bottom lip, an exaggerated look of puzzlement on her face. "Tom Gibbs," she said. "Whatever do you mean?"

"Alice wants you to talk 'sense' into me about Henry and this doctor foolishness. I don't want to debate it now or during supper." Tom snapped open the paper and buried his head in it once more.

Dot smiled and stood up. "There's always tomorrow."

Chapter 3

WITH HER BEDROOM DOOR CLOSED, and a small candle lit on the night table, Alice read Mike's letter. The sewing basket rested wide open on the bed next to her. Tom and Dot's voices could be heard coming from the living room. Despite the distance, Alice caught snippets of their conversation about the government situation, a passionate topic for Tom. Work at the dockyard had been slow all week, and he had come home just as the mailman deposited the mail through the slot in the door. Tom had scooped up the envelopes with a quick glance at the top one before passing them to Alice. "Newfoundland Light and Power," he said. "Seems like bills arrive more frequent than once a month."

Alice spotted Mike's familiar handwriting sticking out from under the bill. "I'll get to these later," she said, and packed them into her sewing basket. Her hand trembled.

The letter lay hidden in the sewing basket all day, nagging at her thoughts, her fingers itching to rip into it. Henry had called to say he would be late. They had decided to wait for him before they ate supper, so she had taken the opportunity to steal away and read the letter.

The glow from the candle cast shadows over the paper as she reread the first line:

I am very proud of Henry, as you must be.

If only Tom felt the same way. Alice's eyes flickered to the door before she continued.

A long-time friend at the university told me in confidence that Henry's been accepted to the medical school. You'll be happy to know he was admitted on the basis of his academic merit along with the endorsement from Dr. Kennedy. The good doctor and my dear friend is highly respected by many of his colleagues who remember him from their time in medical school. Alice, please don't worry about Henry. He'll do fine. My wife and children are anxious to meet my only nephew.

I wish Tom—

Alice became aware the voices had stopped. She dropped the letter in the basket, shut the lid, and snatched her knitting from the bedside table.

The door handle jiggled. Dot moseyed into the room. "So," she said, "what is it?"

Alice stifled a fake yawn. "What do you mean, Mom?"

Dot flipped open the basket and pointed to the letter.

"It's from Mike," Alice said softly.

Dot gently closed the lid. "Henry's home and Tom's wondering where you are."

Alice hid the sewing basket under the bed and went downstairs with her mother.

Henry stood in the front porch taking off his boots. "Sorry I'm late, Mom. Mr. Hull kept me later than I thought."

Dot sucked air through the gap in her teeth. "Doesn't he always? I hope this time you insisted he pay overtime."

"I'll get supper on the go," Alice said. "Tom must be hungry enough by now to chew on the paper."

"Gran," Henry whispered when his mother was out of sight. "How's Dad?"

"Hungry like your mother said. How about you?"

Henry smiled. "Starved."

Dot linked into her grandson. "Onward to the battlefield."

Henry tensed as they approached the kitchen. "Can you stay with us until I leave for university?" he murmured in her ear.

Dot chuckled. "You and your father will survive this little hiccup."

Tom had the table set as he did whenever he had the day off work. Steam spouted from the kettle. He emptied the boiled water into the teapot and placed it on the stove to steep.

Alice smiled and ran a finger along the lid. "It's almost impossible see where you glued it back together."

Dot sat down in her usual place on the inside of the table. "Tom's a handy man to have around," she said. "Alice, my girl, you're one fortunate woman."

Tom remained silent.

Henry pulled out a chair to the right of his grandmother. "Supper smells great, Mom." He looked at his father. "Right, Dad?"

Tom avoided his son's gaze and took his place at the head of the table. His continued silence rang in Henry's ears.

Dot covered Henry's hand with her own. "Jiggs' dinner is a real feast. Mr. Hull planned on ham sandwiches for tonight." She screwed up her face. "For the third time this week."

Tom spread a napkin across his knees. "That's not much of a meal. Especially for the very sick patients."

Alice placed a bowl filled with cabbage, potatoes, turnip, and carrots in the centre of the table followed by pease pudding and chunks of salt meat. "Dig in while it's still hot," she said.

Henry noticed his father spoon every item onto his plate, each movement slow, deliberate.

"You're some quiet tonight, Tom," Dot said. "Something on your mind?"

Alice frowned at her mother.

Henry's heart skipped a beat.

Tom looked his mother-in-law squarely in the eyes. "When I have something to say, I'll say it." His face was calm, relaxed. "I won't need prodding from you or anyone else."

"Welcome to radio station VONF and the Barrelman *show."*

All heads turned toward the radio, which stood on a shelf under the window.

"We Newfoundlanders have a responsibility, a duty toward our children and future generations. Our lives cannot, must not carry on as they have been for the last hundred or more years. How do we go about ensuring a prosperous future that will endure? That is the question which I am certain is uppermost in your minds. I know this, my fellow islanders, because you love this great land with an unrelenting passion."

"The nerve of Joey Smallwood," Alice said. "Telling us what to think."

"Confederation with Canada is the answer, the only answer. The answer that will bring prosperity. Not just prosperity . . ."

Alice chomped on a mouthful of cabbage. "He certainly is long-winded."

Tom chewed a piece of salt meat. The gristle slipped down his throat. "What a load of bull the man's spewing out," he said. "The answer to our problem is to get rid of Commission of

Government. The idea of England making all the decisions about what happens here doesn't sit well with me."

Alice nodded. "It's about time we get back to Responsible Government. We're a separate country and should have the right to run it the way we see fit."

The radio droned on.

"The meeting is at seven-thirty tonight at the CLB Armoury. Come along one and all. Bring your children and learn why Confederation is the only choice that makes any sense. It will be the best thing you'll ever do in your—"

Alice hopped up from the table and tuned the radio to another station. "I can't stand to listen to any more of that horse manure." Static followed before piano music drifted around the kitchen. "That's much better," she said.

Tom went to the stove for the teapot. "Smallwood's wasting his time," he said. "All the man wants is to make a name for himself at this country's expense."

Alice cut up a pan of homemade gingerbread and served it with a dollop of tinned cream over the top. "In my opinion Joey and his co-conspirators are nothing more than traitors to Newfoundland."

Dot looked at the wall clock and caught Henry's eye. "It's seven-twenty. I should get back to the Home."

Henry stared at the gingerbread he'd hardly had time to sample. His mouth watered. "Guess I'll save this for later."

ONLY STANDING ROOM WAS AVAILABLE when Henry and his grandmother arrived at the CLB Armoury. Taller than most of the people there, Henry looked over their heads at the long bench and table set up at the front of the room for Joey and three of his colleagues.

"I want to hear Mr. Smallwood explain how joining Canada has merit," Dot said. "It can't make us worse off than we are right now." A constant hum of voices sizzled the air like an electrical charge. More people packed into the auditorium-sized room, bumping and pushing others into the aisles.

"I hope this meeting doesn't turn angry," Henry said, keeping a protective eye on his grandmother. "Folks get riled up awful easy about politics these days."

"I can't hear myself think with all this noise," Dot shouted.

Henry saw Joey converse with the man sitting to his right. The man smiled, exuding complete confidence. Joey rearranged the papers in front of him then scanned the waiting crowd. He pulled a white handkerchief from inside his suit jacket and cleaned his wire-rimmed glasses with meticulous care. He put the glasses on, neatly refolded the handkerchief, and returned it to his pocket.

Dot tugged on Henry's arm to get his attention. "Let's get closer," she said, and made to push through the crowd. "I want to have a closer look at Mr. Smallwood."

"No, Gran," Henry said, holding her back. "It's safer back here, and easier to get out if anything happens."

Joey drank a full glass of water. "Ladies and gentlemen," he began, his eyes roaming over the people. The deafening hum faded to silence. "It fills me with great pride to see so many Newfoundlanders gathered here tonight. It thrills and excites me. I am overjoyed, but most of all, proud. Proud to see that you have taken a keen interest in this pivotal issue. We will embark on a discussion that will without a doubt change the course of history."

Dot made a clucking sound. "Takes him a while to get 'round to the point. I must admit," she added, "you can't deny he's an eloquent speaker."

Joey hooked his thumbs in his breast pockets, an air of authority about him. “We are a moderate-sized island with a small population. If we continue to stand alone, there is nothing but bleakness ahead.” He paused to look around the room, his gaze fixed from time to time on one person or another. “Poverty will increase. The way of life we treasure above all else will blur into the past.” He paused again. “I have struggled, not for one year, not for two.” His raised fingers to match each number. “Not for three, not even for ten, but for twenty years to find the means to make Newfoundland the best it can be for Newfoundlanders. My friends, Confederation is the answer. Canada is a vast country, a rich country, one that will bestow all its advantages on its newest province.”

“And be Canada’s lapdog instead of England’s!” A man in the front row said.

“You got that right,” the man directly behind him added. “Responsible Government is the way to go.”

Joey raised a steady hand to his glasses, adjusting them more snugly around his ears. “Mr. Jones and Mr. Murphy,” he said, addressing the two men who had interrupted him. “As Canadians, we will have the freedom to govern our province the way we feel will benefit each and every one of us. England has ruled us with an iron fist. Canada will simply guide us with a helping hand.”

A man in his sixties seated in the second-to-last row stood up. “We had Yanks and Canadians here in droves during the war. I for one have had enough of foreigners telling us how to live proper.”

A woman next to him half rose from her chair. “Me and my man can hardly make ends meet with ten youngsters. I say we give Mr. Smallwood a chance to tell us what benefits we’d get if we became Canadians.”

“I was born a Newfoundlander,” a white-haired man

said from the centre of the room, "and intend to die a Newfoundlander, not a bloody Canadian."

Three-quarters of the people applauded.

"I say we listen to what Mr. Smallwood has to say," a young woman shouted over the din. "He makes sense to me."

"You're not much more than a youngster," a deep voice said. "What would you know about politics?"

"She has a right to her opinion," someone else said.

Joey smiled at the young woman. "It is truly heartwarming to see our young taking an active interest in their future. Anyone who strives to hold back Newfoundland is an enemy against hope and prosperity." He directed his attention to the section at his right and honed in on an elderly man with balding white hair. "You good folks know what I mean. Is that not the case, Mr. Edwards?"

Mr. Edwards, a renowned lawyer, stood up. "Mr. Smallwood is a champion for all Newfoundlanders. He has toiled non-stop to . . ."

The back row booed, drowning out the rest of the sentence.

Henry took his grandmother by the arm. "Let's get out of here before a brawl starts," he said, and elbowed his way toward the exit.

Joey spread his arms wide as if to give a blessing. "Is freedom of speech only for those who agree with you?" He spoke in a normal pitch, yet it resonated clearly, audibly. The crowd quieted down.

"I'M VERY IMPRESSED WITH MR. Smallwood," Dot said outside.

"Nothing anyone says or does will make Dad believe in Confederation," Henry said. "He doesn't like any sort of change."

Dot wound her wool scarf more securely around her neck and buried her chin in the folds. "I wish this cold spurt would lift. It makes my skin ache." Arm in arm, she and Henry started up Military Road. They walked along the empty streets where not even a motor car passed by.

"I expect everyone's at the CLB Armoury," Henry said. "Smallwood certainly knows how to keep a cool head. He stopped a near-riot with a few words."

Dot clamped a gloved hand over her nostrils. "I'm sure the hairs in my nose are frozen stiff." She looked at Henry. "I'm surprised Mary Norris wasn't there. She's all for Confederation."

"She knew I'd be there." Henry stared into the distance. "Right now I'm not one of her favourite people."

"She's a thoughtful girl. Let's you know what's on her mind." Dot looked up at her grandson. "It wouldn't hurt to follow her example."

Henry blushed, relieved his cheeks were already red from the biting wind. "Here's Hull Home. Good night, Gran." He turned to leave.

"Hold on a second, Henry. I have one question for you to ponder over tonight."

"What?" he said, wary of what he would hear.

"Did you give Mary any real consideration before you applied for medical school?"

ALICE TOOK MIKE'S LETTER OUT of the sewing box, stuffed it in her pocket, and hurried to the bathroom. Her heart beat faster than her steps. She locked the door, sat on the edge of the cast iron tub, and pulled out the letter. Her eyes scanned the first page again. Footsteps on the stairs caused her to almost slide off the tub. Her breath caught in her throat and she stuffed the letter back in her apron. "Don't be so stunned," she murmured to herself. "Tom can't see what you're doing." When Alice heard the bedroom door close, she retrieved the two sheets of paper, smoothed them out on her lap, and read where she had left off earlier.

I wish Tom would give me a chance to explain why I couldn't make it home for our parents' funerals. It's hard to comprehend that any reason would justify what seems so heartless. I understand why Tom feels the way he does. Still, it's difficult to believe he's this dead set against his son becoming a doctor because of me . . . because of my so-called abandonment of the family. Then again, my brother was always stubborn and quick to jump to conclusions without possession of all the facts. He loves deeply. Unfortunately, he resents just as thoroughly.

Alice, even though we've never met, I feel like I've known you all my life. You want what's best for your family, and would like Tom to at least hear me out. I've decided to come to Newfoundland to face my brother, to urge him to hear what I have to say. I arrive on February 10. Use your own judgment to decide if he should be told about my plan ahead of time.

All the best,
Mike

P.S. Don't you agree the time has come for me to be formally introduced to my little brother's wife?

Alice returned the letter to the envelope, went downstairs to the kitchen, and opened the top cupboard door nearest the pantry. A cookie tin was hidden behind a bag of flour. She hauled off the lid and placed the letter with the many others she had received over the years from Mike. She felt a guilty knot in her stomach at the thought of Tom.

The kitchen door swung open. Alice whirled around. "Henry, what took you so long?" She sounded breathless.

"We were at the big meeting." He took his gingerbread from the oven and sat down.

Alice fidgeted with a button on her dress.

"Mom, I knew you wouldn't be mad at me for going to the CLB Armoury. I did think you'd at least comment on it."

Alice twisted a string around the fingers of one hand until they were all but blue. "Uncle Mike is coming here next month," she blurted.

Henry's fork stopped in mid-air. His mouth drooped open and gingerbread plopped to the plate. "How do you know that?"

Alice bit down on her thumbnail. "Never mind about that now. He wants to settle things with your father once and for all."

Henry laid down the fork. "Dad won't see him, let alone talk to him."

"That's why this has to stay between you and me until Mike gets here."

"When next month?"

Alice squirmed on the chair. "The tenth."

Henry pushed aside the half-eaten gingerbread. "I have an awful bad feeling about this."

Chapter 4

THE SUNLIGHT SPREAD OVER THE houses like a warm blanket, yet when Henry opened the door to get the *Daily News*, the frosty air stole his breath away. He wondered how the meeting had turned out, and saw the answer in big black bold letters sprawled across the top of the front page.

RIOT ALMOST ERUPTS AT CLB ARMOURY

> Tempers flared during the meeting held at the CLB Armoury last evening to discuss the merits of Confederation with Canada. Mr. Smallwood had just begun his speech when several spectators interrupted him to voice their own diverse convictions. Individuals among the crowd then hurled insults at each other, which led to shouting and screaming. Mr. Smallwood remained composed during the incident and managed to control the angry mob. The debate continued in a peaceful manner.
>
> It is this reporter's opinion that Mr. Smallwood

> and his colleagues have a daunting task ahead of them in terms of Confederation. From my personal observations and questioning, our fair city of St. John's is prepared to do whatever is necessary to keep Newfoundland a country. A country proud of its heritage, and most important of all, its independence.

Henry laid the paper in his father's place at the table. "Where's Dad?"

Alice stood at the stove and flipped over a pancake. "He's already eaten and left for work."

Henry snapped open his napkin. "He can't ignore me forever."

"A ship came in last night and has to be unloaded as soon as possible for another trip." Alice put the frying pan in the sink. "You know that isn't unusual." She placed a plateful of pancakes on the table.

Henry watched her smooth butter over a pancake: one, two, three, four, five times. How many more days until Uncle Mike arrived? He caught a sidelong glance from his mother as she smeared a second pancake. The wall clock ticked, ticked.

"Gran asked me to take her shopping on Saturday."

Alice's mouth tilted up in a half-smile. "I think Mom wants to spend as much time with you as possible before you go away." She gave a nervous laugh that sounded like tiny balloons bursting. "Your grandmother has a way about her that will win over your father in the end."

"I doubt even Gran's charms can change Dad's mind," Henry said. "Maybe I should forget about Toronto."

"Get that notion out of your head this minute, young man." Alice stared hard at her son. "You'll be the best doctor to ever practise in Newfoundland."

"I wish Dad felt the same way."

Alice cleared away the dishes. "Get a move on. You don't want to be late for work."

MARY NORRIS TOOK AN ARMFUL of clean bedsheets from the linen closet and started down the hall. She passed the office, the door partly open. Mr. Hull sat at his desk. His wife had all but worn down the carpet from the window to Isaac's desk in the last hour. "Don't tell me not to worry," Mrs. Hull said, her voice a decibel lower than a shout.

Mary scooted behind the door and peeped through the crack.

"Cahill was quite perturbed we hadn't submitted dwelling plans to council," Mrs. Hull continued in a normal tone.

"A mere oversight," Mr. Hull said with the flick of a wrist.

Mary could see the scowl on Mrs. Hull's face when she turned to face her husband. "An oversight that is against the law," she said. "And there will be more trouble because we didn't make applications to become a nursing home."

"No one's bothered us so far with any sort of legalities. It's not like we're operating in secret."

Mrs. Hull flopped into the chair by the desk. "I don't like the idea of Confederation either," she said, her hands palms-down on the armrests.

Mr. Hull's eyebrows drew together. "What does that have to do with us?"

"Things will change. Laws will become stricter."

The jingle of the phone postponed the comment Mr. Hull was about to make. "Hull Home, Mr. Hull speaking. Yes, yes. No problem," he repeated several times during the brief conversation.

"Well, who was it?" Mrs. Hull said in a shrill voice when her husband hung up.

"We may have something to worry about after all." Mr. Hull went to the window and stared outside, his hands deep in his pockets. "The Department of Health and Welfare wants to inspect the Home the day after tomorrow."

Mary gasped.

"Who's there?" Mr. Hull called, heading for the door.

"It's me," Mary said. "I tripped over a bedsheet. Sorry if I disturbed you."

Mrs. Hull shooed Mary away like she was a pesky cat. "Get to work, girl. You're wasting valuable time."

Mary took a deep breath to slow her racing heart before mounting the stairs. At the top she hooked her heel in the carpet runner and stumbled forward. Her shoes came off and the linen fell to the floor. "What else can go wrong?" she grumbled, stooping to retrieve her shoe and bedclothes. Her face drawn, she stomped into Dot's room, changed the bedsheets, pausing often as her thoughts wandered to the imminent inspection. Dot knitted in the armchair by the window in the corner, watching the young woman. Worry lines creased Mary's forehead by the time she had made the fourth and final bed.

"Not even so much as a good morning," Dot said when Mary turned to leave.

Mary froze, stunned, like she had been nabbed in the execution of a criminal act. "I'm sorry, Mrs. Gatherall. I didn't see you sitting there."

"I can see that, child. You look like the sun's about to tumble out of the sky."

"It might be for me." Mary's eyes watered. "I can't handle any more terrible news."

Dot held out her arms. "Come here," she said. Mary approached, and Dot took her hands. "Talk to Henry. He just might put your mind at rest." She squeezed Mary's fingers and let them fall.

Mary tugged on the hem of her apron with both hands. "It's more than that. There's going to be an inspection by the Health Department." She dropped onto Dot's bed. "That can't be a good sign."

MARY BUTTONED HER COAT UP to the collar and put on two pairs of gloves. She pinched her nose to lessen the strong odour of paint which would take at least a week to dissipate. "Night, Mr. Hull," she called down the hallway.

He dumped the last of six oversized cans of tomato soup into a boiler. "Hold on, Mary," he said, and poked his head out the kitchen door. "Glad I caught you. Mrs. Browne spilled a jug of water over her bed. The sheets need changing."

"Right away," Mary said. She fetched fresh linen from the closet and darted to the Annex, happy she had kept her coat and gloves on. The room empty, Mary set about cleaning up. No one to chat with, she completed the task in a matter of minutes. On her way back into the main house, the stench of oil assailed her. She hurried to the kitchen to find it empty. She removed the bubbling soup from the heat before checking the pipes behind the stove. A small patch of oil had collected on the canvas. "Not again," she moaned, and placed a bucket under the leaky pipe. "Mr. Hull!" Her voice blared through the building. "The stove's leaking."

He arrived at her side and gave the area a brief once-over. "I don't see anything," he said. "Mary, girl, you're always on the lookout for problems."

"Can't you smell it?"

"The problem with you is that your nose is too sensitive."

Mary caught a whiff of alcohol under his breath and drew back. She lifted the bucket to show the oil on the floor. "The leak's stopped for now."

"Leave the bucket. If there's any oil in it tomorrow, I'll get the mechanic in."

"Do you think it's a good idea to wait?"

"There's no need to be hasty."

Mary lingered. "Do you want me for anything else?" she said, shooting wary glances behind the stove. "Sheila Vickers wasn't well today. Maybe I should check on her."

Isaac opened a large can of tinned fish. "She coughed up blood a while ago," he said. "I asked young Howard Pike to go for the nurse."

"Poor Sheila. She's only a year older than me."

A gust of Arctic air swirled into the kitchen. "I'm back with the nurse," Howard yelled.

Mary went down the stairs to meet her. "Sheila hasn't eaten since breakfast," she said. "With all the coughing, she came down with a pounding headache."

Jean Baker hung up her coat. "I'll go right on up. Sheila can't afford to miss any meals in her condition."

Mary went back to the kitchen with Howard, the youngest boarder. He warmed his hands over the stove. "Is there any tea ready? It's enough to freeze your fingernails off." He smiled at Mary and the dimples in his cheeks deepened into caverns.

Isaac took several loaves of bread from the pantry. "Supper will be thirty minutes late tonight," he said with a slight slur to his voice. "Mary, butter the bread while I see how Nurse Baker is doing."

"Leave it to him to order you around after hours," Howard

said. He noticed the empty fish cans on the sink counter. "Looks like fish, jam, cheese, and biscuits again tonight. Oh, well, I'm hungry enough to eat anything."

Dot stood to the side of Sheila's bed. Mr. Hull moved around her.

"She's asleep," Nurse Baker said. "She's resting comfortably and her breathing is steady."

Isaac's face glowed like a child given a new train set. "Wonderful news."

"Her temperature's slightly elevated, though." Baker pulled the bedclothes up to Sheila's neck. "I'll stay the night to make sure she's all right."

"Ah . . . Miss Baker," Isaac began. "Is that necessary?"

"I won't expect overtime, Mr. Hull." Baker cooled down the patient's face with a damp cloth. "Since her father passed last year, the poor lass is all alone in the world."

Isaac straightened his tie. "Madam. It's not a question of money. I was merely concerned for your comfort."

Dot moved closer to the bed. "Sheila's been feeling poorly all day, and fell asleep from pure exhaustion." She looked at Isaac. "Maybe Dr. Kennedy should be called in."

Jean smiled. "Don't worry, Mrs. Gatherall. If Sheila shows any sign of distress, I'll call him right away."

"I must get supper ready," Isaac said. He bowed to Dot and lost his balance.

"Oh, my," she said. "Are you all right?"

"Shouldn't turn around so fast." Saliva spurted from Isaac's mouth onto his chin. "Made me dizzy for a second. I'll see you in the dining room," he said, and fled the room.

Dot stared down at Sheila's grey complexion. "Nurse Baker, maybe she should go to the hospital."

"The dear child can't afford it."

"I'll foot the bill for her stay."

"Mrs. Gatherall, it's a kind gesture, but you know very well how proud Sheila is. She won't accept a handout from anyone."

"Well, if she gets worse, I won't give her a choice in the matter."

THE PAPER BOY FLUNG THE *Evening Telegram* to the houses on his route. A paper whizzed by Henry's head, landing on the concrete step. "Great throw, Dougie," Henry yelled at Mary's twelve-year-old brother.

"It's good practice for my slapshot."

Henry picked up the paper from the step and opened the door to the aroma of fried cod. He'd had the meal every Friday of his life, yet never tired of it. He tossed the paper on the couch for his father to read after supper and ambled to the kitchen like he didn't have a care in the world.

Alice placed a bowl of scruncheons on the table and eased into a chair.

"Back trouble again," Tom said. He kneaded the small of her back with one hand. "You've been complaining about that for over a month."

Alice spooned mashed potatoes onto her plate. "It's nothing a little rest won't cure. I've been on my feet all day."

"No more excuses, love. I'll make an appointment with Dr. Kennedy and go along to ensure you show up."

"I have no intention of spending money for no reason at all."

Tom covered his potatoes with mustard. "You're going and that's the end of it."

Alice grabbed up the pickle jar. "We'll see about that," she said, rooting out a cauliflower with a fork.

Henry smiled. He knew his mother would eventually give in. "There's going to be another inspection—" A loud thump on the front door silenced him. His fork landed with a clink on his plate. Tom gaped at his wife. She shrugged.

Footsteps scampered down the hall. Mary hurried into the kitchen, her arms swinging like a sprinter. "Did you read this?" she said, holding out the *Telegram*. She pointed to an article in the newspaper. "There's a detailed report on the Hull Home inspection."

Tom smothered a chuckle. "Not good news, I take it."

Mary sank into the chair next to Alice. She planked her elbows on the table and dropped her chin into her hands. "What am I going to do if the Home closes?"

"Get another job," Henry said. "Mr. Hull would give you a good reference."

Mary punched his upper arm. "It's not that easy. Besides, I love working at Hull Home. I'd miss the residents something terrible."

Alice set a plate in front of her. "Stay for supper. You'll feel better after a full stomach."

Tom's expression became sombre. "What does the report say?"

"It's some awful, Mr. Gibbs. It makes the Home seem like an overcrowded place where everyone is locked away and forced to eat horrible food."

"That sounds about right to me," Tom said.

Alice piled Mary's plate with two pieces of fish, onions, and mashed potatoes. "Mom's never complained about such goings-on," she said, giving her husband a stern look.

Henry picked up Mary's paper and browsed through the report. "It says there's been no dwelling plans submitted or any applications for occupancy or alterations," he said. "All that's required by law."

Mary went ashen. "I overheard Mrs. Hull talk about that."

"Hmm," Tom said. "Doesn't surprise me at all. What else is in the report?"

Mary nearly ripped the paper out of Henry's hands. "The stove should be repaired and a firewall placed behind it. All the exit doors must open out." She read without pausing. "A fire escape or a ramp should be built at the rear of the main building."

"Any mention of problems with the Annex?" Alice asked.

"The hall stove that blocks the door and access to the stairs has to be moved. An exterior staircase is essential and all the chimneys have to be cleaned." Mary whimpered like a small child. "There's no end to these grievances."

Alice smiled at the girl's overwhelmed expression. "They don't appear to be anything too difficult or too expensive to handle."

"Don't raise her hopes," Tom said. "I doubt the Hulls will see it that way."

Mary grew even paler.

"Take heart, love," Tom said in a gentler tone. "Maybe the Hulls will do the sensible thing. Especially with so many helpless people depending on them."

"Of course they will," Alice said. "The Hulls are not stupid."

"I heard some of Cahill and Superintendent Vivian's conversation during the inspection," Mary said. "But after reading what they wrote, I'm scared the Home will close." She lowered her head and played with a slab of onion. "Sorry for barging in on your supper."

Tom raised an eyebrow. "What do you mean, barging in?

You've been welcome here ever since you were a youngster. Now eat up before the fish gets colder than the temperature outside."

A burst of static made everyone realize the radio had been on the whole time. The *Barrelman* show was in progress. Joey Smallwood's voice pealed out like a warning bell. Alice leaped to her feet and switched off the radio. "Mr. Smallwood might as well call it quits," she said. "England will never permit such a ridiculous notion as Confederation."

"I'm not sure about that," Mary said. "Mr. Connors at the Home said England wants rid of us, so they just might go along with it."

Tom shrugged off the statement. "Doesn't matter if they do or they don't," he said. "Newfoundland will always remain a separate country."

Mary licked a piece of crusty fish batter from her lip. "Henry, what happened at the meeting last—" A gentle nudge in the leg caused her to cough.

"What were you saying, Mary?" Tom said when she resumed eating.

"I'm just curious if anyone knows how the meeting at the CLB Armoury went."

Tom sliced through a thick slab of turnip. "Joey and his team harp on about how good a change will be for us," he said. "What's wrong with the ways things are?"

"The way I see it," Mary said, "there's nothing can be done to stop change."

The conversation lulled while they finished the main course. The talk over tea and homemade apple pie centred around the weather, a topic on everyone's mind since the coldest winter on record had struck with an unrelenting hold.

"There's another load of icicles hanging from the roof and

windows," Tom said. "I'd better break them up before they fall on someone."

Alice sighed. "I've never seen the like before this year. New ones appear as soon as the old ones are chopped away."

Mary grinned. "Mr. Gibbs, why don't you wait until they're long enough to slide down to the ground?"

Henry smiled. "Dougie would love that."

"I'd better get to it," Tom said and excused himself. Henry left to put more wood in the grate in the living room.

"That was some good fish, Mrs. Gibbs," Mary said, helping Alice with the dishes. "I wouldn't mind being Catholic if I had to eat fish cooked like that every Friday."

"I wouldn't mind having you as a daughter-in-law, Protestant and all."

The cup Mary was about to put in the cupboard crashed to the floor. "I'm sorry," she cried, and stooped to pick up the shattered remains.

"Be careful," Alice said, bringing out the broom. "You'll cut yourself."

"I'm not always this clumsy."

Alice swept up the mess. "It's only a cup. There's no harm done."

The phone rang. Henry appeared in the kitchen as Alice put the broken shards into the garbage. "Mary, your mother's leaving for bingo in five minutes."

"I need to go now, Mrs. Gibbs. Mom doesn't like to leave Dougie alone in the house."

Henry went with her to the door. "Mom really enjoys your company."

Mary zippered up her rubber boots. "I didn't mean to almost give away the fact you were at the meeting," she said.

"Everything bothers Dad these days."

"I hope things work out between you two."

"Mary, we have to talk about us."

She opened the door. "I need time to think things over." The wind whipped her thick hair around her face as she ran to her house. Henry waited until she was inside to give himself extra time to build up the courage to confront his father. The flames in the fireplace crackled and hissed as he dressed to go outside.

TOM STOOD NEAR THE TOP of the ladder hacking away at an icicle thicker than a man's thigh. Henry darted to the side when the lethal weapon plummeted down. "Dad, I'd like to talk to you about my decision to be a doctor."

Tom's eyes never left the roof. "It won't do any good," he said, the axe held loosely at his side.

"Dad, please."

Tom looked down at his son. "Will anything I say make a difference?"

"No, but—"

Tom swung his arm and smashed the axe into a monster icicle. "Like I told you. It won't do any good."

Chapter 5

THE WIND GROANED AGAINST THE side of the house and rattled the glass in Henry's bedroom window, waking him from a restless sleep. He sat up and stared into the darkness, unsure what had dragged him away from the strange dream. The details bombarded his head, too vivid, too real. He had stood in the kitchen surrounded by his parents and grandmother. His father had pounded the table with a fist. "Mike," he had shouted at Henry. "You've always done what you wanted with never a thought to anyone else."

"I'm not Mike, Dad."

"You're nothing but a selfish bastard."

"Mike," Alice said softly, her eyes sad. "What is wrong with you?"

His grandmother lightly kissed his cheek. "Don't fret none, Henry," she whispered. "It'll all work out." As he turned to her, a thick fog filled the kitchen. Before he had time to call her name, the fog evaporated as if it had never been there. His grandmother was gone.

The plastic sheet over the window bellowed like a balloon

in the Atlantic wind. Through a thin layer of frost he saw a heavy grey cloud swallow the moon, darkening the room until even the shadows disappeared into a black void. Although he hadn't been afraid of the dark even in childhood, Henry tensed. His throat tight, he lay back and tucked the quilts under his chin. No stars. No moon. The bedside clock ticked away the seconds. The plastic sucked in its breath. The glass rattled again. The plastic blew out. In. Out. In. Out. Waiting for air to breathe. Henry couldn't tear his gaze away.

A branch from one of the many maple trees in the yard scraped the window. Henry blinked and looked at the bedside clock. Two in the morning. He rolled onto his side away from the window and closed his eyes. The memory of the dream screamed in his head. Henry turned onto his back and looked toward the window once more. The wind died down. The plastic didn't move. It's stopped breathing, he thought. The clouds separated and the moon's light filtered into the room. The wind stirred again, a gentle breeze at first, then it blew stronger. The plastic ballooned back to life. He closed his eyes and tried to will himself to sleep.

Wide awake, Henry gave up, crawled out of bed, switched on the light, and read from the book he had begun the night before, *The Complete Stories of Sherlock Holmes.* Henry particularly enjoyed Dr. Watson's constant concern for Sherlock's health. Close to four o'clock the book dropped from his hands to his lap as sleep overtook him.

"Henry."

He was certain he could hear his mother call to him. Why did her voice echo like it came from the end of a long tunnel?

His body shook. "Henry, wake up."

He opened his eyes. His mother's hand rested on his

shoulder. He slowly rose his head. "Oww," he said, rubbing the side of his neck.

"That's what you get for spending all night in a chair," Alice said. She picked up the book which had fallen to the floor. "It's a few minutes to nine. Your grandmother expects you at ten to take her shopping."

Henry stretched his arms high above his head to relieve the knot between his shoulder blades. "That won't take more than an hour. Old ladies aren't interested in clothes."

"Indeed," Alice said, smiling to herself on the way out of the room.

Henry dressed in record time and hurried down to the kitchen. His night in the chair had left him shivery all over. He stood by the stove to bathe in its heat. "I don't know how you do it, Mom."

Alice stirred a pot of porridge. "Do what?"

"Get up every morning in the cold to light the hall and kitchen stoves."

"You get used to anything after twenty-five years." Alice removed the cooked porridge from the stove. "Besides," she added with a soft sigh, "your father works hard on the docks in all kinds of weather. He deserves a little comfort to begin the day."

Henry cut bread from a freshly baked loaf and put two slices on the toaster doors and snapped them shut. "You'd have less work if you bought bread from Walsh's Bakery."

Alice turned up her nose. "Baker's fog, you mean. Proper bread is made at home."

The smell of toast filled the kitchen. Henry dished out two bowls of porridge, sprinkled three spoons of sugar on his, and poured in a quarter tin of Carnation milk.

Alice buttered the toast and poured the tea, adding cold water to her mug. "Did you speak to your father last night?"

"I saw him."

Alice looked at her son. He shrugged. She scraped the bowl on a heavy sigh.

"Mom, there's not much time until Uncle Mike arrives."

Alice raised her cup to her lips. "Eight days," she said, and lowered it without tasting a drop of the tea. "You'd better get a move on. Your grandmother will think you've forgotten about her."

DOT WAS DRESSED AND WAITING in her room when Henry charged in. "Right on time," he said. "Told Mom I wouldn't be late."

"I just hung up from her. You must've grown wings and flown here."

Dot linked into him once they were outside and walked to the streetcar stop around the corner on Gower Street. The early February sun reflected blindingly off the snow. Dot shaded her eyes against the brightness. "There's not much heat in the sun," she said. The words were hardly uttered when the streetcar pulled up, almost filled to capacity. They seated themselves near the exit for the short ride to Water Street, the only shopping centre for St. John's and surrounding areas. Henry and Dot disembarked in front of Silver's Jewellery Store a few doors down from the post office.

"Now," Henry said. "Why did you rope me into this shopping expedition?"

"Your mother's birthday is Valentine's Day. I want to buy her a special gift this year. You don't turn fifty every day."

"You always let Mom pick out something."

“She never fails to choose a practical item like an iron. Nothing just for her. Besides,” Dot continued, smiling, “change is good.”

“Tell that to Dad.”

“May I help you, madam?” the tall, thick-chested clerk asked Dot when she laid her purse on the glass countertop.

“Indeed you may. I’d like to look at lockets.”

“Good choice, madam.” He inserted a key into the lock of the glass door on the jewellery display. “We have a wide variety.”

Dot scrutinized over two dozen, seeking Henry’s opinion on each one. “This is perfect,” she said, selecting a sterling silver heart with a straight-line indentation on the front, and plain on the back. The chain measured twelve inches long.

“A wise decision,” the clerk said. “This is one of our recent imports from Switzerland.”

Dot opened the heart. “I’d like a message engraved on both sides.”

The clerk took a pencil from behind his ear and poised it over a notepad. “Go ahead, madam.”

“On the left put ‘Alice, my joy.’” She waited for the clerk to finish writing. “On the right engrave ‘You make me proud.’” She turned to Henry. “One day your father will come to his senses and say the same about you.”

Henry decided not to respond.

The clerk wrote the last word of the inscription. “The locket will be ready on the thirteenth.”

“Grand,” Dot said. “Just in time for my daughter’s birthday. I’ll pay now.” She inclined her head in Henry’s direction. “My grandson will come by for it.”

“Your name and address, sir?” the clerk said, the pencil

once again poised over the notepad. The information recorded, he passed Henry the stub from the envelope containing the locket and chain. "Present this when you come for the locket."

Henry pocketed the stub.

"Now on to Bowring's," Dot said with a satisfied smile. They crossed the busy street to the department store, which stocked every kind of merchandise from the latest fashions to furniture.

Henry trailed behind his grandmother while she browsed through every item of clothing. "Is there anything specific you're looking for?" he said when she crossed the floor to sweaters neatly stacked on a dozen or more shelves.

"Not really."

"I see why you and Mom take hours to buy one thing," he said, hoping to keep any hint of complaint out of his voice.

"You men have no idea what pleasure you're missing out on." Dot moved on to hats, scarves, and footwear.

Henry traipsed along, trying to appear interested. "That's it?" he said when Dot bought the kind of wool gloves he had seen her knit all his life. "We spent hours here for those?"

Dot held out the purchase, a slight grin on her face. "Don't you think they're such a lovely shade of blue?"

"I'm hungry," Henry said. "Time to head out."

"We'll eat here in the Captain's Cabin. I told your mother not to expect you for lunch."

The restaurant, situated on the second floor, was a popular spot for shoppers and visitors to the city, boasting a magnificent view of The Narrows. The entrance to the harbour was bound on both sides by snow-covered, tree-lined hills. A small fishing boat motored out into the ocean. Henry enjoyed the open sea. When he was a boy his father often took him outside The

Narrows to view the whales. He had been ten when he first saw one. The boat nearly tipped over when he jumped to his feet, waving at the whales like they were his best buddies.

A low hum of voices greeted them. Henry spotted Mary seated by a window, a cup clasped between her fingers. She stared down into the wharf. The restaurant was not yet quite full and she had a booth to herself.

His grandmother marched straight for the young woman. "What a pleasant surprise, Mary. May we join you?"

Mary jerked around and gasped at Dot. Her eyes moved to Henry for a few brief seconds before they flickered back to Dot. "Of course, Mrs. Gatherall."

Dot slid into the vacant seat. Henry sat next to Mary. He felt her tense when their thighs touched.

"I pray to God this weather breaks soon," Dot said. She held out her hands, the knuckles crooked and thick. "It's murder on my arthritis."

Mary couldn't quite pull off a smile. "Gramps suffered from it some bad, too."

Henry resisted the urge to hold Mary in his arms.

Dot shimmied out of her coat. "Mary, you look a mite pale. Aren't you feeling well?"

"My migraine's not quite gone. I'll be all right in a while."

Dot rested her back into the cushioned bench. "Thank heavens I don't get them anymore. Now, Henry, I'd like a chicken dinner and a scalding cup of tea. Mary, would you like something to eat?"

Mary swallowed as if the very thought of food was intolerable. "No thank you. My stomach's still off from the migraine."

"Maybe a light soup would help."

"I really couldn't hold down a thing right now," Mary said. "Maybe some dry toast when I go home."

Dot took money from her purse and handed it to her grandson. "Order what you want for yourself. It's my treat."

"He'll pay for his own dinner," Mary said as Henry walked away.

"I know." Dot stared at Mary as if seeking to read her mind. "Dearie, tell me what really troubles you."

"I told you."

"My old eyes have witnessed more sadness and heartache than you can imagine. I recognize terrible worry when I see it."

Mary rocked slowly.

"I know your habits, child," Dot said. "You do that when you're upset or worried."

"The Hulls can be stubborn about repairs. I'm fearful for my job, that's all."

"That's only a small part of it."

Mary's eyelids fluttered as she turned back to the window.

"Love," Dot said softly. "I've known you since you were a baby. I want to help, not pass judgment on you."

Mary slowly turned back to the older woman. "Really, Mrs. Gatherall," she said, wringing her hands. "It's just work."

"Henry's leaving can't be easy for you."

Tears welled in Mary's already red eyes. "Henry doesn't love me enough to stay." She choked off the last word as he approached the table. A hand to the side of her face, she looked away when he sat beside her.

"Mary, are you crying?" When she didn't answer, Henry turned a quizzical face to his grandmother.

Mary looked at Dot. Panic flashed across her drawn features.

"Henry, dear," Dot said. "She misses her grandfather. The loss is still fresh."

Mary dabbed at her tears with a paper napkin. "I must look an awful mess."

Dot slid out of the booth. "Nothing a splash of cold water won't put right. Come along with me, child."

The two women wove their way through the tables, now filled to capacity. Several people noticed Mary's swollen eyes and quickly looked away when she caught them staring at her. Mary hurried on and pushed open the door to the ladies' washroom. Pristine white walls gave the room a sterile hospital look. Water dripped from a faucet in two sinks. A row of mirrors reflected the stalls. The sound of footsteps passed outside, echoing farther into the distance. Relieved no one was there, Mary doused a paper towel with water and wiped her face, plastering strands of hair to her forehead. "I'm a little better now, Mrs. Gatherall." She threw the soaked paper in the garbage container. "I wish Mr. Hull would let me in on what's happening."

Dot smiled at the young woman. "You're not alone," she said. "Never forget that."

"That's very kind of you, Mrs. Gatherall, but I'm all right, like I said." Mary spattered more water on her face and touched up her lipstick. "Please tell Henry I'll see him at work."

Dot combed her hair, washed her hands, and returned to the booth. "Mary's gone home," she said.

Henry hadn't touched his fish and chips. "Gran, she seemed really distracted and I'm sure she'd been crying. Is she honestly that worried about her job?"

"No, Henry. I think it's more than a job."

*

A FULL MOON AND A sky thick with winking stars hung over the city when Henry left his grandmother at Hull Home. After lunch, they had visited all the stores on Water Street and, to Henry's utter disbelief, Dot hadn't bought another thing. Now, anxious to get out of the cold, he walked briskly up Springdale Street to Central Street. The familiar smell of baking bread from Walsh's Bakery gave Henry a sense of comfort and he made a decision. He neared Mary's house and slowed. She hadn't left his thoughts since the Captain's Cabin. She had never been so distant with him, not even in the days following her grandfather's death. He knocked on her door.

Mary answered on the first tap, dressed in boots, coat, and hat. "I saw you from the kitchen window and figured you'd want to talk." She closed the door behind her. "So let's get it over with."

"Why don't we go somewhere warm for a cup of tea?"

"I'd rather walk. The air will help me think clearly."

Henry fell into step beside her. As it was suppertime, they had the street to themselves. They moved in silence, the space between them wide enough for another person. "I told you about applying to medical school," Henry said when he couldn't stand the quiet any longer. "Why are you upset that I've been accepted?" Mary stared ahead. He searched her profile for a clue to her feelings. "Say something," he said. She made no attempt to speak. Henry reached for her. She eluded him and continued to walk. "How do you feel now that I'm leaving for sure?" he said.

"Yes, you did tell me about the decision to apply. But you didn't consult me or ask how I felt about it."

"I hoped you'd be happy for me."

Mary turned to him, her eyes ablaze. "Did you give any thought to me or to our future together?"

Henry looked down at his feet. "I grabbed at this one chance to make something of myself. I couldn't, can't think about anything else."

Mary took a few steps toward him. "You'll be away for at least eight years. What am I supposed to do in the meantime? Twiddle my thumbs? Read? Or would you rather I pine after you like a lovesick schoolgirl?"

"We . . . we'll sort something out."

"Be serious, Henry. I'll be close to thirty years old by the time you're done. There's a right good chance you'll meet someone else." She slumped, drained of energy. "Besides, I don't want to be sorted out."

Henry's mouth opened but no words came out.

Mary sighed. "I went out with someone a full year before you. When you and I made love you were well aware it was my first time."

"I don't get what you're trying to say."

"Really, Henry. Then allow me to explain." Mary moved even closer to him. "You've known me my entire life. I'm not a casual person. I believed we were committed to each other, intended to spend our lives together."

"You make it sound like I played with your feelings, used you."

"Think about it, Henry. One way or another, isn't that exactly what you did?"

Henry wanted to say something, anything, but he couldn't get his tongue to function.

Mary stood tall. "Don't worry. I won't stand in your way."

"Mary." Henry reached out to her. She shrugged away from

his touch. “We have to talk about this.” He didn’t recognize his own voice.

“Everything isn’t always about you, Henry.” Mary pushed past him and ran back to her house.

Henry stared at her, his face whiter than the snow which had just begun to whirl around him.

Chapter 6

MARY STARED OUT THE BEDROOM window as night gave way to day. The stars, which had dotted the sky like silver sparkles, had faded. White, fluffy clouds glided slowly, waiting for smaller clouds to catch up. Mary blew out her breath and watched it transform into a grey mist. The smell of bacon drifted into her room. Her stomach growled, yet the thought of food chased away her appetite.

Light footsteps ran down the front hall and her mother's voice chimed through the house. "Dougie, don't forget to put on your cap. It's extra nippy this morning."

Dougie had delivered the morning *Daily News* and Mary heard the front door slam when he came in. She scrunched into a ball and covered her head.

"No need to shake the whole house," she heard her mother mumble on the stairs.

Mary closed her eyes to fight back tears.

Her mother came into the room. "Love, you're not up yet. Are you under the weather?" She took hold of Mary's chin to study her face, the way she had done when Mary was a child.

"Where'd those dark circles come from?"

"Mom, I'm worried Hull Home might have to close."

"You're whiter than new bedsheets. It must be more than that."

Mary lifted the quilts from her like it was a delicate operation and rolled over to the side of the bed. She held onto her head. "I have another migraine. The pain's so bad I can't see straight."

"Stay put. I'll bring you up a cup of hot tea and call Mr. Hull."

"That's not necessary, Mom."

Flora produced one of the sad smiles that had become the norm since her father's passing. She kissed her daughter's cold cheek. "One day's loss of wages won't send us to the poorhouse."

"Really, Mom. My head's not bad enough to miss work."

Flora's hand flew to her mouth. "Oh, dear me," she said. "It just occurred to me you're upset about Henry."

"He's not the only man in the world," Mary said.

"Love, denying your true feelings won't make them go away."

Mary rocked to help cope with the drumming in her head, which radiated down to her shoulders. The bed creaked. "I can't think about anything right now, Mom."

Flora went to the door. "I don't mean to preach, but running from the truth helps no one," she said with a crack in her voice. "Breakfast is ready. Don't be long."

Mary opened the night table drawer and took out a picture of her father. He looked up at her, a mischievous glint in his eyes. A tear splashed onto the glass and slid down to the wooden frame. She tossed the photo back in the drawer and slammed it shut. Her head almost exploded from the loud thud.

*

SCRAMBLED EGGS, BACON, HAM, AND tea awaited Mary when she went downstairs. She succeeded in keeping down a piece of ham.

"You'll get sick if you don't eat," her mother said when she pushed the food away.

Mary drained the tea in one gulp. "Mom, you know my stomach's always off with a migraine."

Flora picked up the phone by the side of the fridge. "1590 M please," she said.

Mary spun in her chair to look at her mother. "What are you doing?"

Flora held a hand over the mouthpiece. "I'm calling Mr. Hull to tell him you're sick and won't be in today."

Mary took the phone and cancelled the call. "Mom, I told you I'm all right. Anyway, the fresh air will do me good.

"Promise me you'll eat something when you get to the Home."

"I will," Mary said.

She bundled up with an extra scarf wrapped around her nose and mouth. Within seconds the air penetrated the woollen material, drying her mouth and stinging the back of her throat. A heavy snowfall overnight made walking more difficult. Her headache dulled to a tolerable throb. People merely nodded as they plodded by, eager to reach their destinations and bask in precious warmth. Grey clouds gathered, darkening an already gloomy day. Mary arrived at the Home and promptly put on a pot of tea. She toasted one slice of bread to quell her nausea. Her stomach churned even more at the first nibble.

Dot strolled into the kitchen. "How are you today?" she asked, her eyes on the toast Mary had hardly touched. "Still don't have much of an appetite?"

"Has Mr. Hull brought up the inspection to you?" Mary said, lowering her voice.

"I see you're not ready to admit what's really troubling you," Dot said. "That's fine for now." She looked down the hall. "By the way, there's no need to whisper."

Mary's face relaxed. "Mr. Hull doesn't like me to meddle in his business."

"If the Home closes it will matter to us all." Dot poured a mug of tea and took a sip. "Mr. Hull's not spoken a word to me. He doesn't appear worried either." She moved the cup back and forth between her hands. "With what was printed in the paper, I'd be a little more anxious in his place."

Mary nibbled at a corner of the dry, crusty toast. "Is he here?"

"Stayed all night again. He made breakfast and left when he received a call from his wife."

Mary stopped chewing. "She's gotten bad news about the Home!"

"Not at all," Dot said. "Mrs. Hull has the sniffles and wanted Mr. Hull to fetch some cough syrup." She chuckled. "Mrs. Hull demands immediate attention."

Nurse Jean Baker entered the kitchen wearing an extra sweater. "The rooms are hard to keep warm in the winter," she said, taking two mugs from a rack on the sink counter. "I don't want Sheila Vickers to catch pneumonia on top of tuberculosis. Hot tea and toast will do the trick."

"How is she?" Mary asked.

"Dr. Kennedy stopped by earlier to see her. He's pleased with her progress."

Dot retrieved a tray for the nurse. "The poor darling wants to be home by Easter."

"That isn't likely to happen," Jean said. "She'll be here until Christmas for sure."

Dot placed milk and sugar on the tray. "Susan enjoys mystery books. I'll go by the library to take out a few for her."

"She'll appreciate that," Jean said, and left with the tray loaded down with tea, gingersnap cookies, and toast.

"Now, Mary," Dot said once they were alone again. "Did you get an opportunity to talk to Henry?"

Mary rinsed her cup. "Yes. I told him to go to Toronto and not give me another thought."

BY NOON, MARY HAD SCRUBBED the upstairs hallway in the main house and made all the beds, including those in the Annex. She found it easy to avoid Henry, as he rarely left the office. Her stomach had settled down by one o'clock. The hunger pangs which had gnawed at her all morning drove her to the kitchen. She hadn't packed a lunch and helped herself to a bowl of the tomato soup simmering in an oversized pot on the stove. She crumbled a handful of salted crackers into the thick red liquid. The first taste burned the tip of her tongue. She blew on the next one before gingerly putting it into her mouth.

Mary slurped at the last dregs of soup in the bowl when Mr. Hull returned. "Good afternoon," she said. "I hope your wife is doing better."

Mr. Hull passed the table without a word or a glance at Mary. He stirred the pot, his eyes glued to one spot on the wall.

Mary stood up. "Mr. Hull. Are you all right?"

He turned around. "Oh. Mary. I didn't see you there." Soup dripped from the ladle to the floor. He didn't notice even when several drops found his shoe.

Mary carried her dirty dishes to the sink. “Is anything the matter?”

“Not a thing,” Mr. Hull said, resuming the task at hand.

Mary wiped crumbs from the table. “I’ll see if the residents are ready for dinner.”

Mr. Hull opened a loaf of baker’s bread. “Good idea,” he said, again not looking at her.

Mary glanced back at her employer as she left the kitchen. He swayed slightly and stirred the pot with both hands as if the soup resisted his efforts. “He’s acting some strange,” she murmured under her breath on the way to the dining room at the far end of the hall. Many of the residents had assembled for dinner, their voices buzzing as they waited for the midday meal to be served. The walls were white, the top half covered with striped green wallpaper. Lighted by a single light bulb in the centre of the ceiling, dark green curtains were pulled wide open on the large side window. Dot and two other women occupied a table set for four. Mary sat down next to Dot.

“Mary,” the woman across from her said, “what’s the soup for today?”

Mary produced a crooked smile. “Tomato, I’m afraid.”

The woman groaned. “That makes five days in a row.”

“Oh, well,” the tiny woman next to her said. “At least it’ll be nice and hot.” She pulled her cardigan more snugly around her thin waist. “It’s cold enough in here to wear long johns.” Her teeth chattered.

The two elderly widows continued with the soup conversation, giving Mary the chance to speak in private with Dot. “Mr. Hull seems a tad out of sorts.” She bent close to Dot. “I had the impression he was tipsy.”

“He does like a nip or two every now and again.”

"Has he heard back from City Council or the Fire Department?"

"As a matter of fact—"

"I knew it," Mary said, cutting across her. "He has to correct all the violations, doesn't he?" She babbled on. "He'll close down rather than spend all that money."

Dot wagged a finger in front of Mary's face. "You need to give up that habit of always leaping to hasty conclusions," she said. "He merely received a letter from the city stating they weren't aware he operated a nursing home. That's all."

Mary twirled strands of hair around her forefinger. "Why go to the trouble of an inspection if they don't intend to enforce the recommendations?"

"That's City Hall for you," Dot said.

Mary gazed around the dining room. "That does it," she said. "They have the power to close the Home."

"Child," Dot said. "What a thing to say. They wouldn't put sick people and old folk on the street in this weather."

Mary pushed back the chair and rose to her feet. "Don't bet all your savings on that. I'd better get to the kitchen before Mr. Hull has a fit," she said, and bustled away.

A round old woman with thin white hair sat at the table drinking tea. "Hello, love," she said as Mary came in.

"Oh, hello," Mary said, taken aback. "Are you here to see a resident?"

"No, I came to see Mr. Hull. A friend of mine told me he charges three cents cheaper a day than the government's old-age home." She smiled. Dimples formed in her wrinkled cheeks. "I move in here tomorrow morning. Every penny counts."

Isaac breezed into the kitchen. "Indeed it does, Mrs. Hayes," he said with a light step. "Indeed it does."

MARY SAT IN DR. WHEELER'S spacious waiting room and looked around at the unfamiliar area. Twelve chairs lined three walls, and a children's wooden table and chairs occupied a corner. A supply of blank paper and crayons rested on the shiny red surface. In the centre, burdened with stacks of magazines, stood a mahogany coffee table. Mary glanced at the cover of one magazine; a smiling woman was making a cake for a freckled-faced boy. He knelt on a chair poking a finger into the batter as his father walked through the door with an even bigger smile than his wife. She pulled out another magazine from the pile. More images of happy family life. Mary threw down the magazine.

A man in his seventies sat on the other side of the room. Two seats down from him was a woman with a boy of about ten or eleven. The boy's runny nose never quite cleared despite constant wiping. His cough—a hacking sound deep down in the bottom of his lungs—eased occasionally. The receptionist, the man, and the woman were engaged in a discussion about Joey Smallwood's campaign to join Confederation.

"In my opinion," the woman said, "the man's on a mission to destroy this beautiful land. I heard talk there will be a vote soon to decide."

"Good," the receptionist said. "That'll put an end to this nonsense once and for all."

Mary gripped her purse tighter.

"I doubt that," the woman replied. "Mr. Smallwood's very passionate about Confederation. He won't give up until he's won."

The man turned to her. "I'm afraid you're right on that score, young lady." He shook his head as if to prepare his listeners for bad news. "I have friends from around the bay who swear that most of the outport communities are all for Confederation. They think Mr. Smallwood knows what's best."

The intercom on the desk buzzed. "Yes, Doctor," the receptionist said, then showed the woman and child into the office. Mary browsed through a travel magazine, her gaze constantly straying to the clock over the desk. Three o'clock. She promised Mr. Hull to be back by three-thirty. He would dock her pay for the extra time missed. She glanced at the clock again. The minute hand slithered forward.

The boy and his mother came out of the office. "You're ever so kind, Doctor," the woman said over her son's cough. "I can't thank you enough for the medicine."

Dr. Wheeler, a man well into his sixties, waved the thanks away. "It's not doing anyone any good sitting in my cabinet." He turned to the old gentleman. "Your turn, Mr. Gough."

The receptionist smiled at Mary. "It won't be much longer," she said. "Mr. Gough takes no more than a minute or two."

True to her word, the man had exited the office by the time the boy and his mother had put on their coats.

"Go right in," the receptionist said to Mary.

An overwhelming desire to close out the world anchored Mary to the chair. She wished she could be anywhere else. Her palms were clammy when she seated herself before the doctor.

"What brings you here today, young lady?"

"I . . ." Mary paused and lowered her eyes.

"Come," Dr. Wheeler said softly. "My new patients soon learn there's nothing they can't tell me."

Mary looked up, her eyes moist. "I have awful bad headaches and feel like vomiting all the time."

"How's your appetite?"

"Food turns my stomach."

"Let me examine you and find out what's going on."

A plump nurse led Mary into a room off the office. The white-sheeted examination table conjured up an ice-covered lake ready to crack open and drown her. The stirrups belonged to a horned monster eager to trap her in its grip. The colourless, lifeless walls were harsh, sterile.

The nurse passed her a gown. "Put this on," she said with a cheery voice. "The doctor will be in presently."

Mary's fingers trembled as she took off her clothes and sat up on the table.

A slight tap on the door made her jump. "This won't take much time," Dr. Wheeler said.

Mary lay back and stared at the ceiling. Her fingers dug into the sides of the table's mattress.

"I understand you're worried," the doctor said. "Try to relax."

Mary closed her eyes as the doctor probed every inch of her. She tried to imagine sitting in front of a roaring fireplace.

"All done, Miss Norris. I'll see you in my office when you're ready."

The nurse helped Mary into a sitting position. "Now that wasn't so bad," she said.

Mary shivered even though the room was warm. She tried to put on a smile but couldn't muster one.

DR. WHEELER FINISHED WRITING IN Mary's file when she returned to his office. "I'm afraid the news may not be what you want to hear."

Mary squished her hat into a tiny ball between sweaty hands.

The doctor closed her folder. "We have to do more tests, of course. Once those are done, we'll discuss your options."

The pain behind Mary's eyes intensified. She saw double.

ALICE WALKED TOWARD DR. KENNEDY'S surgery. She had convinced Tom to stay at work and not fuss about her. Alice increased her speed and saw Mary come out of a building at the end of the road. She called to her. Mary pressed on, lost from sight by the time Alice reached Dr. Kennedy's house.

"Good afternoon, Mrs. Gibbs," the receptionist said. "Lucky for you we're not busy today."

Alice smiled at the only other patient, a man her age she didn't know. She leafed through a magazine about institutionalized care and only looked up when the man was shown into the office. Her back began to hurt.

"Your turn, Alice," Dr. Kennedy said in his professional voice.

Alice slowly rose, a hand gripping the small of her back. Once she straightened up, the pain eased enough for her to hurry into the office.

"Looks like arthritis has settled in," Dr. Kennedy said after a brisk prodding of her spine and lower back

"I was afraid of that," Alice said. "Dad suffered from crippling arthritis. He ended up in a wheelchair."

"Your father was diagnosed with severe arthritis in his early twenties." The doctor smiled. "Your symptoms are milder and associated with aging."

"Tom will be glad to hear that."

"Is he still angry with Henry?"

Alice slumped back in the chair. "Henry might as well be a boarder for all the attention Tom gives him these days."

"Have you told him that Mike's coming?"

Alice stared, then smiled. "I should have known he'd write his closest friend."

"He'll be staying with me," Dr. Kennedy said. "He wrote that you would decide whether to tell Tom or not. I take it you haven't."

"He'd go out of his way to avoid Mike. I won't take that chance." Alice moved a fraction to alleviate the dull knot in her back. "He'll be some mad with me when he finds out I kept it from him." She put her elbows on the desk. "He'll be put off that you gave me Mike's address."

"I'll risk that," the doctor said. "Tom is a reasonable man, yet when it concerns Mike he becomes a different person."

Alice picked up her purse from the floor. "Tom won't speak to Mike."

"Maybe he'll give in when he's face to face with him."

Alice sighed. "Do you really believe that?"

"Tom wouldn't stay this angry after all these years if he didn't still love his big brother."

Chapter 7

TOM TRUDGED THROUGH THE FRESHLY fallen snow on his way home from work. Every muscle in his body screamed from hours of unloading heavy crates from the cargo ship. He pulled his coat collar up to cover his ears. The wind whipped snow, which felt more like chips of ice, into his eyes. He tugged his salt-and-pepper hat down over his forehead and jogged the last few yards to his house. Baby icicles jeered at him from the edges of every window. "You won't win over me," Tom said, and hurried inside. The smell of meat roasting in the oven and a wave of heat welcomed him.

"I'm home," he called, and sat on the hall chair to untie his boots.

Alice's voice drifted toward him, humming "Let Me Fish Off Cape St. Mary's" in the soft, sweet tone she had used on Henry when he was a baby. He paused to listen, sure she could have been a professional entertainer if she had wanted. A sadness he hadn't heard before resonated from every word. Boots placed on the mat to dry, Tom went into the kitchen. A light whirl of steam rose from a gingerbread loaf cooling on the sink counter.

"Hmm," he said, breaking off a considerable chunk. "There's nothing tastier than gingerbread with tinned cream."

Alice whacked his hand with a spoon when he reached for another piece. "Save some for the rest of us." She donned an oven mitt and pulled open the oven door. A lock of her hair blew in the heat.

Tom moved next to her. "Ah, that's feels good," he said. "Too bad we can't heat up the docks like that."

Alice lifted the lid from the roaster. The juice hissed and popped like a summer hail shower on asphalt. "I didn't expect you for another hour," she said.

"Some of the men complained they couldn't feel their toes, so we were let go early."

"You have to go back after supper then?"

"There's not much left to do."

Alice basted the meat, closed the oven door, and tweaked her husband's nose. "That's redder than beet juice, not to mention colder than an ice cube." She reached up to the cupboard for plates. "Ow!" she cried, grabbing hold of the sink counter. "My arthritis is some bad today."

Tom took down three plates. "This weather's not much help either."

Alice pressed a hand to the small of her back. "I asked Mom to supper. She's coming with Henry."

Tom placed an extra plate on the table. "I'll go shave before they get here." He scratched the stubble on his chin. "You take it easy. I'll set the table when I'm done."

"Hold on a minute," Alice said when he turned to leave. "I want a word with you while we're alone."

"Can't it wait?"

"Do you want to be a part of Henry's life?"

"I'll get aspirin from the bathroom for you," Tom said.

"I'm waiting for an answer."

"Of course I want to be a part of Henry's life. What kind of question is that?"

"A reasonable one considering you've hardly spoken to him since his acceptance to medical school. If it keeps up you'll push him away for good."

Water boiled out of the kettle spout and sizzled on the stove. Tom snatched the handle and moved it to the back of the stove.

Alice put on the remaining oven mitt. "Are you going to answer my question?" She bent forward to get the roast from the oven. "Oh, God," she cried. "I can't straighten up."

Tom grabbed a dishcloth and took the roaster from her. "Let me get that aspirin for you."

"Don't try to change the subject, Tom Gibbs. Henry's going whether you approve or not."

"He's made it clear he doesn't need my approval," Tom said, and walked out of the kitchen.

HENRY COPIED DOWN NUMBER AFTER number into the accounts ledger, yet one number stuck in his head. Two. Mike would arrive in two days. He yawned.

Isaac glanced up from the papers on his desk. "You look more tired than I feel," he said. "It's five-thirty. High time you were off."

Henry threw down his pen and shut the ledger. "I was supposed to meet Gran in the entrance a half-hour ago."

"You're right about that," Dot said. She stood in the office doorway with hands on her hips. "I had half a mind to go on without you." The phone rang. "That'll be Alice wondering where we are."

Isaac picked up the receiver. “They'll be there shortly, Mrs. Gibbs. And by the way, I didn't ask Henry to stay late.”

“For a change,” Dot mumbled as she turned to leave the office.

“Sorry, Gran, I've been preoccupied all day,” Henry said from behind her. He took his coat from the hook. “Have you seen Mary?”

“She brought supper over to Sheila Vickers in the Annex.” Dot shot him a quick look. “Did you want her for anything special?”

“I haven't had a quiet talk with her in days.” Henry buttoned up his coat lopsided.

“Something is distracting you,” Dot said, fiddling with his buttons.

Henry sighed. “I want to make sure Mary's all right.”

Dot took off her gloves. “I'll wait in the entrance while you drop over to the Annex. Only an idiot puts off important business.”

“Promise I won't take long,” Henry said, and scurried to the Annex. He met Mary at the bottom of the stairs, hedging around the hall stove.

“Your grandmother's not in her room,” she said.

“I wanted to see you.”

“You shouldn't keep Mrs. Gatherall waiting any longer.” Mary stepped around Henry. “I'm much too busy to talk.”

Henry blocked her path. “I really thought you were all right with me applying for medical school.”

Mary held his gaze. ”You really do have a high opinion of yourself.” She sighed as if bored. “Do as you please. I don't want to talk about it.”

The door opened. Icy wind chased Mr. Hull inside. “Mary,

for goodness' sakes, what's the holdup? You should have the soup on the dining room table by now."

"It's my fault she's late," Henry said. "I kept her talking."

Mary left without a word to either man.

"She's not herself lately," Mr. Hull said with a shake of the head. "This is the second time today I had to go look for her."

"Mary is probably suffering from another migraine," Henry said. "The smell from the oil paint is still some strong."

Mr. Hull smiled at Dot on his way back to the kitchen. "Have a good evening," he said.

"I tried to delay him from spoiling your chat with Mary," Dot said when she and Henry were at the streetcar stop. She rolled her eyes. "It would've been easier to get a day-old infant to waltz. Did you get a chance to find out what's on Mary's mind?"

Henry looked down at his grandmother. "To tell the truth, Gran, I'm more confused than I was before."

The wind churned up the snow and sprinkled it over their faces. Henry thought his lungs would crack like an eggshell if he breathed in too deeply.

Dot sneezed three times. "The air has a bite like a hungry wolf," she said, pinching the bridge of her nose to ward off another sneeze.

"Maybe we should catch a taxi," Henry said, and waited for the usual objection.

"I am feeling stuffed up," his grandmother said.

"You must really be under the weather." Henry hailed down a car. Dot insisted she would pay the driver, but Henry paid the fare plus tip before she could open her purse.

The taxi man tipped his salt-and-pepper cap to them. "Have a good night, folks."

Dot hurried inside. She went directly to the kitchen, leaving on her winter attire. "I'll never be warm again," she said, huddling close to the stove. Snow melted into a puddle around her boots.

Tom took her coat and placed a shawl around her shoulders. "The Home never seems to quite warm up, does it?" he said.

"Thank you kindly, love," Dot said, sitting down at the table. "That's much better."

When everyone had dug into the meal of meat, turnip, carrots, and gravy, Tom grinned at his mother-in-law. "I wonder what's for supper at the Home?"

"Look here," Dot said in a voice that belied the stern expression on her face. "You ask the same question every time I come over. I'll give the same answer as usual. Canned fish, fruit, cheese, and toast."

Tom folded a slice of bread in two. "You forgot biscuits." He smacked his lips together. "Sounds delicious. Are you allowed jam with the toast?"

Dot heaved an exaggerated sigh, pretending to be annoyed. "Yes, Tom. We're allowed jam. Before you lecture me about the food at the Home like you always do, it's not that bad." She turned to her daughter. "I have to admit your daily visits with leftovers lend a bit of variety."

"Dot," Tom said, "there will always be a room here for you. And," he added, "you'd be company for Alice."

"I knew you'd get around to that sooner or later."

"Don't waste your breath, Tom," Alice said. "Mom won't leave Hull Home."

Dot patted away a drop of gravy from the corner of her mouth with a napkin. "Actually, I've been giving that some thought these past few weeks."

Alice gaped at her mother. "You've been so adamant about the Home. What's changed your mind?"

"I'd love to have a room to myself again." She looked at Tom with a sheepish expression. "To be honest, I am kind of turned off from canned fish and tomato soup."

"Grand," he said. "We'll stop by for your belongings tomorrow."

"I'm paid up to the middle of the month. Wait till then."

TOM LEFT HOME AT SIX the next morning, the early dawn dulled by cloud cover. Alice's back had bothered her most of the night. He had crept out of bed without disturbing her when she had finally gone to sleep. He reached the waterfront where other longshoremen were already gathered to begin work.

A middle-aged man came up behind Tom. "Days like this are cold enough to freeze your socks off," he said. "I reckon you wish you'd stayed at Newfoundland Margarine all those years ago." His breath vaporized with each word.

Tom bunched up his shoulders against the weather. "Sure do, Bill. A comfortable office would be some nice right now."

Bill's face lost its humour. "My weary bones won't be able to take this strenuous work for much longer."

The two men looked toward the cargo ship from Canada, which had docked an hour earlier, low in the water with the load of food and clothes. "This one will take all day to unload," Henry said, sighing inwardly. "Maybe into tonight and tomorrow as well."

The foreman called from the end of the wharf. "Tom! Bill! The sooner we start, the sooner we get out of this cold."

The specific tasks assigned, the men got under way. Bill and several others brought up crates from below deck. Tom hooked them onto the crane to be lowered to the wharf. The crates were then hoisted onto trucks to be delivered all over the island. Mid-morning, a heavy snow fell. The men took a tea break to warm themselves and waited for the weather to clear. The snow tapered to a light dusting and work resumed.

Bill handed Tom a crate of winter coats. "We should get extra pay for working under these North Pole conditions."

Tom chuckled. "I'd say you're too old to be a dreamer."

Bill flexed his fingers. "They're stiffer than a starched shirt collar."

The sun came out as the morning wore on with little effect on the temperature. "One more crate to load and we can go to dinner," Bill said on his way below deck.

Tom removed a glove and reached into his pocket for a clean handkerchief. About to blow his nose, an odd grinding noise caught his attention. The hair bristled on the back of his neck. He looked down to the wharf. The men had stopped working. They stared up at him, waving their arms like puppets, shouting. He couldn't make out a single word. Tom glanced behind him. Nothing unusual. He turned to the right. Everything normal there, as well. He stared down at the men once more. They pointed, their faces white. The grating, strained sound grew louder. Closer.

Tom whirled around. A large crate spun out of control, twirling like a spin top, bearing down on him, mere feet away. He snapped his head in every direction. Nowhere to run. No protection. The crate swooped nearer, hungry to smash into his body.

"God help me," Tom whispered, and leaped over the side of the ship. A crate whizzed by and crashed, crumbling into shreds of wood and broken dishes.

Bill bounded up from below deck. "Tom, what in God's name made that racket?" He looked around for his partner. "Tom. Where are you?" He blessed himself and scrambled over the debris to the side of the ship.

The men on the wharf stood motionless, a prayer on each pair of lips.

The taste of blood and the crunch of bone were the last Tom knew before the world blackened around him.

BILL RAN INTO THE OFFICE at Hull Home, panting, clutching at his chest.

Henry almost vaulted over his desk. "What's the matter, Mr. Bartlett?"

"Henry," Bill said between gasps. "An . . . accident . . ." He doubled over to get air into his lungs.

Henry felt weak all over. "Is it Dad? Has he been in an accident at work?"

Bill collapsed into a chair. "They brought him to St. Clare's Hospital."

Henry gave him a drink of water. "Is he badly hurt?"

Bill paled under the redness caused from exhaustion and windburn. "He looked awful bad. I came straight here from the wharf."

"I'll get Mom," Henry said, halfway out the door.

"Don't worry about her," Bill said. "I'll see your mother gets to the hospital."

Henry sprinted the short distance to the hospital, his coattails flying behind him. He found his mother all alone in the waiting room, her eyes red and swollen. A light over her head dulled then brightened, repeating the pattern a second time, not sure whether to die out or stay on. Alice looked in his direction. The light dulled again. Her face became lost in the gloom. Henry's stomach lurched. He wanted to run away, to hide from the words he feared would destroy his world. "Mom," he said instead, sinking into the seat beside her. "How's Dad?"

She reached for his hands and laid them on her lap. "All I know for sure is that he's still alive."

Henry fell back in the chair with relief. "Who told you about Dad?"

Tears tumbled down Alice's cheek and collected under her chin. A few splashed onto Henry's hand. "Dr. Kennedy heard about the accident and drove me here. We arrived the same time as the ambulance. Your father was unconscious." Alice gripped her son's hands so tightly her knuckles turned white. "His face and jacket were drenched with blood."

"Mom, it mightn't be as bad as it looked. Head wounds, even ones that aren't serious, bleed a lot."

Alice gave no indication she heard her son. "Mike didn't make it home for his parents' funerals." She stared past Henry, her eyes glossy. "He will be home for his brother's funeral."

"Mom, look at me. You have to believe that Dad will be all right."

"Life's funny. Tom survived four years in the Great War only to be killed at work."

Henry shook his mother by the shoulders. "Stop talking like that. Dad's strong. He'll be home in no time."

Alice caressed his cheek with the back of her hand. "Love," she said, "the crane broke while it was hoisting up a huge crate. Your father had to jump from the ship all the way down to the wharf to avoid being crushed."

"Oh, my God!" Henry cried.

"That's like jumping from the roof of a four-storey

building." A sob escaped her lips, tightly pressed together. "No one could survive that."

"Tom Gibbs did," Dr. Kennedy said. He rolled down his shirt sleeves.

Henry's mouth went dry. "H-how bad is it?"

"Both heels were crushed in the fall."

Alice stared at the floor. "There was so much blood."

"I've never met a man as lucky as Tom," Dr. Kennedy said. "He had a severe nosebleed. The longshoremen who witnessed the fall said when Tom hit the ground feet first, he rolled and struck his nose against the posts along the edge of the wharf."

Henry put his hands under his legs to keep them from shaking. "Dad's all right?"

"Yes," the doctor said. "He'll be laid up for a while with his heels, but apart from two black eyes and a broken nose, he's grand."

Alice stood up. Her purse dropped from her knees to the floor. "Can I see him now?"

"He's being cleaned up. I'll be back in a few minutes to take you in."

Alice sat down again. "I must make my face presentable before I see your father." She pulled a handkerchief from her purse. "He'll be some upset if he thought I was bawling on his account."

"I just thought of something," Henry said. "Dad will have no choice but to listen to Uncle Mike."

Alice drew her eyebrows together. "Why?"

"He won't be able to walk away."

"Sweet Virgin Mary, you're right," Alice said. "That will only make him madder at us for not warning him."

Chapter 8

ALICE TROD SOFTLY DOWN THE stairs, dressed in her nightgown and housecoat, relishing the heat from the hall stove. Eggs frolicked in bacon fat, bread toasted in the toaster, and tea steeped on the stove when she walked into the kitchen. "It's lovely to have someone else light the stoves and make breakfast once in a while," she said, planting a kiss on her son's cheek.

Henry turned over the eggs. Fat flicked on his thumb. "You look awful, Mom," he said, sucking the inflamed flesh. "Didn't you sleep?"

"It was some hard to close my eyes without your father next to me." Alice made tea for both of them. "It's only six-thirty. Seems you didn't get much sleep either."

"It's the tenth, Mom. Don't you remember what that means?"

"Mike's due today," Alice said. She sat down and tasted her tea. "I've thought about nothing else for days."

Henry placed two plates of greasy eggs and toast on the table.

"Thanks, love," Alice said. "Your grandmother says that

thinking good thoughts will make good things happen." She cut the egg into small pieces. "It can't hurt to give it a try."

"Gran always sees the best in everything," Henry said with a wistful smile.

"God bless her," Alice said. "I don't know what I'd do without her."

Neither spoke as they ate . . . or tried to. A quick succession of even beats on the front door pierced the silence. Alice knocked her cup over. Tea flowed across the table and dribbled over the edge. She pushed back her chair in time to escape staining her housecoat. "Good heavens! That can't be Mike already?" Henry scrambled away from the table and hurried to answer the door. Burned rubber assailed his senses.

Dougie stood on the concrete step. "Look, Henry," he said, pointing toward New Gower Street. "A fire!"

Dark grey smoke billowed up, blackening the blue sky. "It looks like Horwood Lumber," Henry said.

Alice stood next to her son. "I don't think so," she said. "The fire seems farther down than that."

ISAAC HULL HAULED OUT HIS chain watch from his pocket as he left the Annex, and walked across the backyard to return to the main building. Six-fifty. He was late getting breakfast under way.

Mary rushed toward him. "Mr. Hull, there's smoke coming from behind the stove and from under the kettle."

"It's probably nothing serious," Isaac said. "You go check on Sheila Vickers. She coughed something fierce while I was lighting the coal stove."

Mary wrung her hands. "But Mr. Hull, nothing like that ever happened before. We have . . ."

Isaac disregarded her and made for the kitchen. Suddenly, flames surrounded the stove and licked at him, spreading along the ceiling. Isaac started for the sink to get a bucket for water when flames jumped across the space to the counter. "Goodness me," he yelped. After one more half-hearted attempt, he turned and fled.

Howard Pike ran out of the dining room. "Mr. Hull," he said in a high-pitched tone. "We have to help the residents get out."

"Call the Fire Department," Isaac said, and zoomed past the boy. "Fire!" he shouted, running down the stairs for the front door.

Howard snatched up the hall phone receiver and dialled the operator. Sweat bubbled on his forehead as the fire bore close to him. His shirt stuck to him like he had been caught in a rainstorm.

"Number please," a female voice said.

"Hull Home's on fire!" Smoke curled around Howard. "Hurry," he coughed. Flames crept along the wall and began to eat the wire connected to the phone. Static sizzled in Howard's ear.

"I'm sorry," the operator said. "Please repeat . . ." more static.

"Fire at Hull Home," Howard shouted. "Call the fire—" The wire melted like black licorice. He dropped the phone. Smoke stung his eyes as he stumbled toward the stairs, groping along the wall. "Fire," he tried to yell, but his voice cracked. He spit out the charred taste of smoke and tried again. A croak came out.

Hands out, probing, Howard found the stairs. He inhaled smoke with every breath. He covered his mouth with the tail end of his shirt and climbed two steps. Water streamed down his soot-stained face, his lungs struggling to take in air. His head spun.

"Is that you, young Howard?" Joe Oliver, the oldest resident, yelled from above.

"Yes, Mr. Oliver. I'll get you out."

"Don't come up here, lad. You'll get yourself killed."

A wave of flames shot down the stairs, forcing Howard back. "I'll get help, Mr. Oliver," he said. Exhausted, he crawled on hands and knees to the exit.

Mr. Hull raced from the sidewalk and dragged him to a safe distance.

"It's like the fire of hell in there," Howard said. "The poor residents won't stand a chance if we don't help."

A fully equipped Bickle fire truck rolled to a stop in front of the Home. Like a well-choreographed dance routine, District Chief Baker and six firemen leaped to the ground with an easy, practised movement, each man in tune with the other. They dislodged hatchets, unloaded the two ladders, and unwound the hose with grace and efficiency. "How in God's name did this happen?" the chief said to no one in particular as he assessed the building. Flames burst out through all the windows on the eastern section. Four elderly men cowered together in the top flat window. "Get the ladders on the building, boys," Baker ordered. "Call in the central fire station. We need all the help we can get."

A wiry, bent old man hung a leg over the window ledge.

"Good Jesus," a bystander said. "He's going to jump."

The ladder slapped against the side of the house. A fireman raced up the rungs like a black widow spider. "I got you, old-timer," he said. "You're safe now."

Low murmurs rippled through the crowd as the fireman bought each man down. Two more firemen tried to enter the building through the front door to no avail while erratic spurts of water sprayed the burning building. “The fire’s everywhere,” the oldest firefighter reported to Baker. “And the hose is frozen to the ground.”

A Bickle fire truck from the central station skidded to a stop on the black ice. Baker quickly apprised Chief Cadigan of the situation. “I’ll take care of the Annex,” Cadigan said, and signalled his men to get out the hose for the other building.

Three windows on the second floor blew out, one after the other. Slivers of glass showered down like hail on the people below. “Move back,” Baker instructed the crowd.

A hunched-over woman dressed in a nightgown appeared in a corner window. “The hall’s filled with fire,” she cried. “I can’t get out of my room.”

“Hold on,” Baker said. “We’ll get the ladder to you.”

“It’s too late,” the woman screamed, fire snapping at her heels. She crawled onto the window ledge and jumped. The tail of her green nightgown glowed yellow with fire. Three men ran to the building and held their arms out to catch her.

Baker ran over. “How is she?”

One of the men cradled the woman to his chest, her head turned up to him. He blessed himself and gently closed her eyes.

Fire Superintendent Vivian pushed through the crowd. He gazed down at the remains of the old lady, a blanket draped over her broken form.

MRS. DUGGAN SAT UP IN bed. The room looked unfamiliar, then she remembered Mr. Hull had asked her to move the night before. A putrid smell had awakened her and she now realized it was smoke. She sidled to the edge of the bed, her arthritic knees cracking. Fatigue acquired from long months of tuberculosis hindered her progress. The door seemed far away, a pinpoint on the horizon. She staggered close enough to reach out and turn the brass knob. The stench of fumes and intolerable heat knocked her back. The roar of fire travelled up the stairs. She looked at her husband's picture next to the bed.

The sounds of voices from the street led her to the window. She picked up a vase from a side table and bashed out the glass.

"Jump," Isaac and Howard shouted to her in unison. "We'll catch you."

"I'll get Mrs. Lamb to the window first." She roused her roommate from a deep sleep.

"W-what's the matter?" the blind woman asked, groggy, disoriented. "Is that smoke I smell?"

Mrs. Duggan's voice trembled. "The Home's on fire."

Mrs. Lamb folded wrinkled hands under her chin. "Our Father Who Art in Heaven," she prayed.

"Come with me, Mrs. Lamb. We have to go out the window."

"Hallowed be Thy Name, Thy Kingdom come," the frail voice continued.

Mrs. Duggan tugged on her arm. "Please, Mrs. Lamb, come on."

Heat from the fire pressed against the door. It rattled, held strong for a few seconds, then burst open. Thick, black smoke rolled over the two women, and Mrs. Duggan's throat constricted. She gasped for breath and slumped over Mrs. Lamb's lifeless body.

In the next room, Joan Parsons, a woman of fifty, heard a cry for help and bolted out of bed. Smoke curled around her head. She gagged. Flames rose up outside the window. She woke the three other patients and ran across the hall to the room at the front of the Home. Firemen below beckoned to her. She ran back to her room. "The window in the other room is clear of fire. We can get out that way."

"No," one woman wept. "I'm afraid."

"We're better off waiting here," another said.

Joan glanced at the flames licking the window. "Don't be so stunned. We'll die in here." The three women clutched each other and wouldn't budge. Joan hurried back across the hall and threw up the window.

"Jump," the crowd yelled. She crawled onto the ledge and looked toward the sky. "Sweet Jesus, protect me," she said, and let herself go. Three young lads broke her fall. One set of young hands broke loose from Joan's weight and her left hip smacked the sidewalk with a sound like the crack of a whip.

Another window exploded on the third floor. A man jumped. People slipped on the ice and tripped over each other in an attempt to catch him. The thud when he hit the ground stilled the crowd. Even the wind seemed to quiet down in respect for the crumpled body of the old gentleman on the cold, hard sidewalk, a look of terror in his wide, sea-green eyes. One of the several Salvation Army members who had come with hot tea and blankets gently placed a soft white quilt over him.

A mattress emerged from a second-storey window, followed by a wail sharper than the cold. No one appeared in the window.

"Captain," a fireman said to Baker, "the smoke and heat's keeping us from going in through the windows."

"Come with me," Baker said, and went to the back of the building with Superintendent Vivian in tow. Two women lay side by side on the ground, both wrapped in blankets. One moved. One didn't. Baker knew the latter was dead before he touched her. He smiled at the woman who looked up at him, her cheeks stained with soot, her eyes wide with fear. "Don't worry, ma'am, we'll get you to the hospital." He faced his crew. "Inside, men," he roared. "We can't allow any more of these good people to die."

They broke in the door and bounded up the stairs through smoke as black as night and heat intense enough to scorch the hairs on their hands. The lead man tripped over a stout woman half sitting against the wall. He felt for a pulse. "She's alive," he said. The superintendent and Baker slung her over the fireman's shoulder.

"Help me," a weak voice said from the first room on the left. A tiny, thin man was sprawled over a bed. The mattress caught fire as he was lifted up.

Baker went back into the hall. Unable to reach any other room, he cupped his hands around his mouth. "Is there anyone here?" The floor groaned and creaked under his feet. Vivian pulled him to safety the same instant the boards buckled and gave way.

"Captain," the fireman carrying the old man said. "There's nothing more we can do here."

"All right, men, outside."

They dodged sudden outbreaks of fire, sidestepped fallen debris, and fought through dense smoke, emerging from a heat wave into a frosty bite. "Keep the hoses on the Annex," Baker ordered. "The fire doesn't seem to have taken as much of a hold there." He took off his fire helmet and ran short, thick fingers through wet hair plastered to his scalp. "At least those residents will have half a chance."

MARY RAN INTO THE BACK room of the second floor in the Annex. Mr. Bartlett had a suitcase open on his bed. "You don't have time to pack," Mary said, taking his arm and urging him toward the door.

The old man looked at her as if she had sworn at him. "I'm not going anywhere without my belongings," he said, and trotted to the bureau.

"Look around you, Mr. Bartlett. There's smoke everywhere."

"All right, all right." He took his suitcase and followed Mary out of the room.

They came to Sally Cranshaw's room. "Come with us," Mary said.

"I won't leave without my cameo brooch." Sally's bony fingers shook as she searched the top drawer of the bureau. "My grandmother gave it to me over seventy years ago."

Mary sent Mr. Bartlett ahead. "Mrs. Cranshaw, we don't have time for this."

Sally kept fumbling in the drawer.

"Stand back," Mary said through gritted teeth. She pulled the drawer out and dumped the contents on the floor. The cameo landed at her feet. "I'll hold onto it for you."

"Thank you, Mary, but I want to keep it with me."

"The smoke is getting thicker," Mary said. "We must go." She took Sally's hand and headed for the stairs. Mary retched, covered her mouth with her apron, and forced the bile back down her throat.

Smoke floated around them, denser than thick fog. Sally gripped the rail. "I can hardly see a thing. Oh, Mary, we're not going to make it out alive."

"Nonsense," Mary said in a strong voice. Her eyes stung, her tongue felt too big for her mouth, and her lungs burned. She bumped into the stove at the bottom and guided Sally around it. She tried the door. "It's stuck," she said, pulling on the handle with both hands. "I have to go back upstairs for the others, Mrs. Cranshaw." She spit out grey saliva. "You keep trying the door."

The old lady kicked the door. "I'll get this nuisance opened if it's the last thing I do."

Mary summoned up a reserve of strength from somewhere deep inside and sprinted up the stairs two at a time to find Dot directing residents down the hall to the stairs in an orderly fashion. She smiled at Mary. "My John was in the army and taught me to keep a sensible head in times like this."

"I'll go help Sheila Vickers," Mary said.

A fluffy cloud of smoke smouldered near the ceiling in the sick girl's room. She sat up on her elbows. "I was some scared, Mary. What's happened?"

Mary pulled the covers off Sheila. "The Home's on fire."

Sheila dragged one leg at a time over the side of the bed. "I'm some tired, Mary. I don't think I can walk."

Mary helped her stand up. "Lean on me. I won't let you fall."

Sheila's legs wobbled like wooden wheels, but they made it into the hallway. Mary handed her over to Mr. Connors, a male boarder. "Don't you worry none, lass. I'll get Sheila out in one piece."

A sound like wind howling came from overhead. "The fire's in the roof," Dot said. "Please God it doesn't cave in before we're all out."

Sally appeared at the top of the stairs, knelt down, and searched the floor.

"Good God," Mary moaned. "What's she doing back up here?"

"I dropped the brooch," Sally said. "It's all I have left in the world."

"Mary, get her downstairs this minute," Dot said. "I'll look for the brooch."

Mary lifted Sally to her feet and guided her back down the stairs. "You have to promise to stay here this time," she said.

Mr. Connors winked at Mary. "I'll see that she does." He pulled at the door handle. "I don't suppose the damn, blasted thing is locked."

"Not when I came over," Mary said, and tracked her way back to the second floor. At the top of the stairs, Mary vomited. Grey-black smoke swirled and gushed along the hall like water through a tunnel, washing over her, coating her face and clothes. She threw up again. "Mrs. Gatherall," she called to the shadowy lump near the floor. Mary coughed. Her saliva had dried up. "Did you find the brooch?" Her words were mere squeaks. Mary fumbled through the haze down the hall. The shadow lay face down, a cameo rested between the fingers of the right hand. "Mrs. Gatherall?" Mary felt for a pulse. She tried to yell but no sound came out.

A noise like the brakes of a train smothered Mary's attempt to cry out. She looked up. The ceiling sagged, fractured like a broken eggshell. Mary held a hand to her abdomen. *I'm sorry, little one.* The roof moaned one last time and plummeted. If Mary screamed, no one heard it.

Chapter 9

ALICE AND HENRY WENT BACK into the kitchen to the distant clink of fire bells. "I wonder where the fire is?" Alice said. She refilled their teacups.

"Maybe we'll hear something on the radio," Henry said, switching the button to the on position. An unfamiliar tune—a happy song about singing in the rain—blasted into the room.

"Can't be that big a fire, then," Alice said.

"We only saw smoke," Henry said, taking a sip of tea. "Maybe the firemen will get it under control before there's too much damage."

The song faded out and the announcer's voice came on.

"And now for the seven-thirty news. A building is burning in the downtown area with flames shooting twenty feet into the air. Two people have died in the blaze. Firefighters from two stations are battling below-zero temperatures, freezing water, and blinding smoke to evacuate the building. Traffic is at a standstill and the police are advising everyone to take an alternate route to work. We'll keep you updated as more information becomes available."

"How terrible," Alice said. "I hope it doesn't spread up our way."

Henry ate the last of his breakfast and was about to leave for work when the radio announcer came on. "*We've just learned that the fire is at Hull Home, the nursing home on the corner of Springdale and New Gower Street.*"

"Mom!" Alice cried. "Oh, God, Henry!"

"I'll go see if she's all right."

Alice hurried down the hall behind him. "I'm coming with you."

"No, Mom. Wait here. I'll call you as soon as I find Gran."

Henry flew down the street. Flakes of ash floated in the air, mixing with a light flutter of snow. Two dead. The words were imprinted on his brain. Could Gran be one of them?

Mary.

His heart thudded like horses' hooves on concrete. He tried to push the dark thoughts away. They persisted, pushing forward, tormenting, as the wind roared past his ears. Cold sweat dried on his chilled body. "Mary has to be all right," he muttered. A burst of guilt knotted his gut. "Gran, too," he said over and over. His breath condensed into clouds which didn't have time to evaporate before he ran through them.

The crowd thickened the closer he came to the Home, slowing him to a crawl. Black smoke, a grey sky, and the sun—now a ghostly shadow—witnessed his progress.

Henry shoved past two men. "The poor souls," he heard one say.

"How many dead?" the second man asked.

"I heard it's at least twenty."

Henry drove himself harder. He reached New Gower Street and threaded through the onlookers until he reached the Home. Mr. Hull and Howard Pike stood on the sidewalk outside the Annex. Bodies lay in a row on the sidewalk, covered with blankets. Henry stared at them in disbelief. He had to find out if Mary and Gran were among them.

A firm hand clamped down on his shoulder, pinning him to the spot. "Sorry, son," Fire Superintendent Vivian said. "You can't go near the bodies."

"Mary works here." Henry tried to wriggle free from the vicelike grip. "My grandmother's a resident."

Howard ran over to Henry. "Mrs. Gatherall's still inside," he shouted over the din of voices, traffic, and spraying water. His face was blackened with smoke, his eyes bloodshot. Tracks of sweat left smudges on both cheeks. "So's Mary."

Henry stopped struggling with the fire inspector. "Let go of me. I'm going inside."

"I can't allow that, son," the inspector said. Henry summoned every ounce of strength and pulled free.

Howard caught up with him at the door to the Annex and clutched at his arm. "Don't be so stunned, Henry. You'll only get in the firemen's way."

Henry jerked away. "I have to do something."

A hacking cough sounded close by. Howard and Henry looked toward the Annex. Mr. Connors came through the door with Susan Vickers in his arms, followed by a clump of residents, the weaker ones assisted by firemen.

Henry looked past them. "Mr. Connors, where's Mary and Gran?"

"They were getting everyone out of bed the last time I saw them."

Susan clung to Mr. Connors, her nightgown black and torn. "Oh, Henry." Her chin quivered. "Mary stayed behind to help us." Another coughing fit seized her, shaking her whole body. Mr. Connors continued with her to the table where the Salvation Army handed out blankets, hot tea, and words of encouragement.

Alice stumbled out from among the bystanders. "Henry, I can't find Mom."

Susan Vickers made a noise, nothing more than a whimper from a dry and scorched throat, yet loud enough for Henry and Alice to turn and see her look at the Annex.

Two firemen walked from the building, a limp form held in each man's arms.

Henry caught his mother as her knees buckled like an accordion, her breathing fast, hard. He felt her heart pound.

"Please God," Alice whispered. "Mom has to be alive." She looked into Henry's eyes. "It's all right. Let me go."

Dot's head rested against the fireman's chest. One arm hung loose and swayed with every step he took. "I'm sorry, ma'am," he said, and placed the body on the ground. Alice gathered Dot in her arms. She stroked her mother's hair, rocking her like a baby.

"Gran," Henry mumbled. No time for tears. His grandmother would want him to do what was important: look out for the living. The second fireman placed a young woman on a blanket. The wind blew hair away from her face. "She looks some peaceful," he said. "You wouldn't know but she's asleep."

A Salvation Army man draped the body with a blanket, sighing as he pulled it over her head.

All Henry could do was stand and stare.

"I have a daughter about her age," the fireman said. "Do you know her, young man?"

Henry nodded. "Her . . . her name is Joan Myers. She was due to go home next week after spending eighteen months at the Home. She was some excited." He summoned every ounce of stamina to remain on his feet. "For a second, I thought she was . . . someone else."

"I hope you find your friend," the fireman said, and turned to leave.

Howard snagged him by the coat. "Wait, sir," he said. "Mary Norris is still in there." He looked at Alice. "She was with Mrs. Gatherall."

"Higgins," Chief Baker said to the fireman. "Go make sure everyone stays a safe distance back from the Home." He took off his hat and wiped his arm across his forehead. "Lads," he said, addressing Henry and Howard. "We've been through the entire building. I'm sorry. There's no one left inside."

"She must be in there," Howard said. He gaped at Henry. "I didn't see her come out. Where else can she be?"

Henry stared at the Annex, his face a blank. "I need to go in and make sure," he said.

"That's out of the question," Captain Baker said.

"Henry," Isaac Hull shouted as he made his way over. "Mary was brought out earlier."

"Is she all right?" Henry looked all around. "Where is she?'

"The ambulance took her to St. Clare's. The ceiling fell in on her." Isaac didn't look directly at Henry. "And on your grandmother."

Henry heard the words, garbled like they had been filtered through a sea of water.

"You go to the hospital," a female voice said. "I'll meet you there later."

More distorted words. Henry turned in their direction.

"Henry?"

He blinked.

Alice stared up at her son. "You go to the hospital," she repeated, and looked back at her mother. "I'll be there soon."

Henry knelt beside his grandmother. "I love you, Gran," he said, and kissed her forehead.

"Let me tell your father about Mom," Alice said. "You know how fond he is . . . was of her."

TOM WOKE TO THE NOISE of the breakfast trolley squeaking down the hall toward his ward. He tried to sit up, and only succeeded by digging his elbows into the mattress and dragging himself against the bed-head. His heels throbbed, his head ached. Every muscle twitched and rebelled at the slightest movement. The trolley squeaked closer. Tom's nose itched. He nearly cried out in agony when he scratched it.

"I know exactly how you feel," the man in the next bed said. "A broken nose isn't any fun." He tapped the side of his. "Mine's been broken four times."

Tom looked out the window. "The sky is thick with smoke," he said. He tried to get a better look, but drab curtains blocked his view.

"Must be a fire," his neighbour to the left said.

"Seems like the smoke's down around Water Street," someone observed.

A nurse laid a tray on Tom's bed trolley. "Hull Home has all but burned down to the ground," she said.

Tom jerked forward. His heels pushed into the bed and the pain knifed up his legs. "What!" he said. "Was anyone hurt?"

The nurse glanced out the window. "I'm afraid so. Over twenty people are dead by last count."

The chatter around the room stopped.

Tom pushed the bed trolley away and threw off the bedsheets. He threw his legs over the side of the bed, grunting all the while.

The nurse looked at him, her lips puckered. She said nothing.

When his legs finally dangled like trousers on a clothesline, the nurse spoke. "Now, Mr. Gibbs, where do you think you're going?"

"My son works at the Home."

"You plan on dragging yourself there by the arse?"

Tom glared at her. "If I have to."

"It's only just gone eight," the nurse said with a calm that unnerved Tom. "What time does he start work?"

"Eight," Tom barked. "Why do you—" Tom went limp with relief. "Thank God. He would've been at home when the fire began."

"There you go. He's safe."

Tom stiffened. "Oh, no. My mother-in-law lives at Hull Home."

"I'm awful sorry to hear that," the nurse said, hoisting Tom's legs back onto the bed. "But there's nothing you can do for her. Which building was her bedroom in?" she said as an afterthought.

"The Annex. Why?"

"A speck of good luck for you. Most of the survivors are from the Annex."

Johnny Hayes, the young man in the corner bed, switched on his radio. The song "Jack Was Every Inch A Sailor" was just ending. "My grandmother moved from the Sanatorium to Hull Home a few days ago."

"The Hull Home fire is under control. The thirty-four confirmed dead are being transported to the General Hospital for autopsy. Our next song is dedicated to all the mothers and fathers who perished in the tragedy."

"A Mother's Love Is A Blessing" began to play.

The nurse handed out the last tray. "Everyone eat up or you'll have me to answer to," she said from the doorway. "That's a threat, not a promise."

"Mrs. Dwyer is some good nurse," one man said after her departure. "Though I wouldn't want to rub her the wrong way."

A few faint chuckles quickly died away.

HENRY CRACKED OPEN THE DOOR to Mary's private room and peeped inside. He had begged the nurse to tell him how she was. She couldn't do that. He wasn't a family member. "I'm going out with her," he had insisted, but that wasn't enough. Henry stared at her, dumbfounded. "How is love measured?" he said, and walked toward the stairs. As he climbed to the third floor, all he knew for certain was that Mary was still alive.

Henry took several deep breaths and pushed open Mary's door once more. The room was in darkness, the sun hidden behind black, smoke-filled clouds. If only he could hide away from his pain, his mother's pain, Mary's pain. Everyone's pain.

Mrs. Norris sat at the bedside, humming a soft lullaby to the inert figure on the bed, a mere shape under a blanket. She turned when a shadow fell over her. "Hello, Henry," she said softly, dabbing her eyes with a tissue.

Henry opened his mouth to answer but remained silent when he saw the equipment hooked up to Mary.

"She needs oxygen to help her breathe," Mrs. Norris said quietly, repeating the doctor's exact words. "She's suffering from smoke inhalation." Mrs. Norris sighed and reached for her daughter's hand. "Her lungs may be permanently scarred."

Henry took a step forward. Mary's face was lost in shadow. Tubes coiled around the bed, snaking up her arm to her face. She didn't move.

"The roof collapsed on her. She has a broken shoulder and a severe concussion." Mrs. Norris kissed her daughter's hand. "My sweet girl may have brain damage."

The world's gone crazy, Henry thought. His chest tightened. "When will they know anything?"

Mrs. Norris let go of Mary's hand and slumped back in the chair. Her arms drooped by her side. "She has to wake up before they can do any tests."

Henry held his breath and moved closer to the bed. He said a silent prayer, then gazed down at Mary. Soot and perspiration streaked her face. A bandage encircled her head. Clotted blood smeared her forehead and matted her long hair.

"I don't want Dougie to see her like this," Mrs. Norris said. She covered her mouth to hold back a sob.

Henry touched Mary's cold cheek. "Please, Mary," he whispered. "Don't leave me."

Chapter 10

MIKE CLOSED THE BOOK HE hadn't been able to concentrate on and tugged the straps of the seat belt around his waist. The flight had been long, with too much time to weigh out the possible outcomes of his visit. He hadn't allowed himself to do that before. The closer the plane cruised toward Newfoundland, the more his resolve faltered. Too late to turn back now. Restless, he sighed, knowing he couldn't give up, even if it were possible.

Tall and broad-shouldered like his younger brother, he had been cramped in a space not meant for a man his size. The metal lock clicked into place. The same sound echoed throughout the compartment. All seat belts secured, the plane tilted to the right on its approach to the airport. Mike looked out the window at the birthplace he hadn't seen in forty years. He felt something wet on his cheek. He brushed it away. The plane passed over The Narrows and the harbour lined with the Portuguese White Fleet, the group of fishing vessels so named because they were all painted white. A huge cargo ship was in the process of being unloaded. Tom was probably one of the longshoremen unloading the merchandise.

Mike leaned his head back against the seat. Tom had been a mere boy of ten when he left. Would he recognize the man he had grown into? A sense of loss overpowered him, a physical ache in the pit of his stomach.

"You've gone rather pale," the elderly man next to him said. "Are you all right?"

"Yes," Mike said. "Just a lot of regrets floating around in my head."

"I left Newfoundland sixty years ago," the old man said. "And come back for a visit every chance I get." He smiled. "It's best to leave regrets in the past and focus on happy memories."

Mike closed his eyes. How many happy memories had he missed out on? He had missed Tom's graduation from school, his marriage. Missed the birth of his only nephew. Missed time together as brothers.

"SIR?"

Mike's eyes flew open.

The stewardess leaned over him. "All the passengers have disembarked," she said. "Do you require assistance?"

"No, thank you," Mike said. He put on his coat and followed the young woman to the front of the plane.

"Have a pleasant stay," she said.

"Goodbye," Mike said, and descended the steps to the asphalt. The winter air nipped at his skin like a pickaxe. Inside the terminal he collected his luggage and called a taxi.

"Home for a visit, are ya?" the driver said when Mike gave him the address.

Mike sat forward. "What makes you think I'm from here?"

"Well, now, buddy." The taxi man glanced in the rear-view mirror at his passenger. "The way you talk is a dead giveaway."

"That's one less thing Tom will have to criticize," Mike murmured.

"What was that, buddy?"

Mike took off his hat and laid it on the seat. "I've been away for forty years."

"You still have family here?"

"A younger brother and his family."

"He must've been a youngster when you left."

"Tommy was ten."

They passed alongside Quidi Vidi Lake. Mike looked at the ice-covered water. "I rowed in the Regatta three years in a row," he said. "They were good times."

"The record's still not broken."

Mike heard a hint of pride in the man's voice.

"My father was the skip of the winning crew," the driver continued. "I rowed myself for a while. The body's not up for it anymore."

A grey haze hung over the city. "As the plane was coming in for a landing," Mike said, "I saw clouds of smoke in the downtown area. Know anything about that?"

The taxi man gave a shrill whistle. "An awful fire first thing this morning. Never seen anything like it before in all my days. Water from the hoses froze into monstrous icicles the second it touched the building. Some of the firemen were treated for frostbite." He paused. Mike waited for the driver to continue. When he did, his voice vibrated with a touch of sadness. "That wasn't the worst part." He shoved his hat back from his eyes. "Thirty-four people died. I still can't fathom it."

"What caused the fire?"

"Don't know as yet."

"Where was the fire?"

The driver pulled up in front of Dr. Kennedy's house and the question was lost in the sound of the brakes. "Here we are," he said in a livelier tone.

Mike paid the fare and stepped onto the sidewalk with two suitcases.

"Need help with the luggage, buddy?'

"Thanks. I'll manage."

"The sidewalk's like glass. Mind you don't fall down."

Dr. Kennedy hurried out, having thrown his coat on when he saw the taxi stop. He pulled Mike into an embrace. "I meant to meet you at the airport, but I'm not long home myself."

Mike smelled smoke on his clothes. "That's a doctor's lot in life for you." He noticed the doctor's drawn expression.

Dr. Kennedy lifted the larger suitcase from the ground. "Let's get inside where it's warm and cozy. It must feel strange to be back."

"You can't imagine." Mike looked around at the homes painted red, green, and yellow. Signs of uniqueness and character, as far as he was concerned.

The doctor looked his friend up and down. "You look good, considering . . ."

Mike smiled. "Considering we're old men." He retrieved the remaining suitcase from the ground and trod with caution across the shiny snow.

SEATED IN FRONT OF A roaring fire in the library, the two enjoyed hot tea. "We'll have something a bit stronger later," the doctor said. He shivered, even though the room was stuffy with heat. "Right now I need a clear head to get my thoughts in order."

"It's wonderful to see you after all these years, Frankie," Mike said. "You've hardly changed."

"No one's called me that since my Charlotte passed." He stared at nothing in particular. "Medical school was quite a while ago." He looked at Mike with a whimsical spark in his eyes. "And I had a full head of hair then." The fire crackled. "Life twists and turns us into places we should never have to go."

"Sometimes we aren't given a choice," Mike said.

Dr. Kennedy laid his mug down and pulled on a bushy eyebrow. "We have a lot to talk about, Mike."

"I see old habits never die. It's a wonder you have any eyebrows left."

Mrs. Simms, the housekeeper and cook, stuck her head in the door. "Dinner's ready, Dr. Kennedy. Salt fish with drawn butter, like you asked. Would you be wanting me to serve it now?"

"Yes, thank you, Mrs. Simms."

"Mmmm," Mike said. "Haven't had that since I left."

The doctor stood up, his stooped shoulders now more pronounced, and led the way to the dining room. They sat at the long, dark table decked out with a linen cloth, china dishes, and silver cutlery. Carnations set in a white porcelain vase graced the centre. Dr. Kennedy chuckled. "Mrs. Simms has gone all out for you." A Persian rug covered most of the hardwood floor. A wedding portrait of Dr. Kennedy and his wife hung over the marble mantel. Candles glowed from either end.

"Charlotte was quite beautiful," Mike said, taking note of her auburn curls and rosy complexion.

"Indeed she was." Dr. Kennedy sighed.

Dinner conversation was sparse, confined to the weather and how much the city had developed over the years. Dr. Kennedy wolfed down the food while Mike picked at his.

"Which is it?" the doctor asked.

Mike looked up, startled, as if surprised to find he wasn't alone. "What?"

"You're not hungry or you don't like Mrs. Simms's cooking?"

"This is more delicious than I remember."

"Then eat up. Mrs. Simms expects you to clean the plate." The doctor lowered his voice as if to inform his friend of a possible conspiracy. "She won't let you have any homemade coconut cream pie if you don't."

"We wouldn't want that," Mike said, and proceeded to eat every morsel.

The meal over, the doctor showed him to his room. "Come down to the library for a drink when you're ready."

Dr. Kennedy sat, elbows on the armrests of the chair, and swished brandy around in a glass when Mike joined him. A bottle of brandy and another glass stood on the table next to him. Mike half filled the glass, sat in the same armchair as before, threw back his head, and downed the drink in one swallow.

"It's been one hell of a day," Dr. Kennedy began without looking at his guest. "A most regrettable couple of days, to tell the truth."

"I heard about the fire. Where was it?"

"Hull Home, a combination boarding and nursing home."

"Isn't that where Henry works?"

"The blaze began a few hours before he started work. I knew all the residents, Mike, administered to their medical needs, listened when they cried." The doctor fell back into his chair. "I've never felt so useless, so unnecessary, as I did today."

"The darker side of our practice," Mike said.

"Tom's mother-in-law died in the fire. He thought the world

of her. She risked her life helping others make it to safety." The doctor paused when the flames in the grate sputtered. "Henry's girl, Mary Norris, is in serious condition."

Mike poured another drink from the bottle of brandy.

Dr. Kennedy held out his glass for a refill. "There's something else I haven't told you." He took a swig of the drink. "Tom had an accident at work."

Mike's glass rolled across the hardware floor to the fireplace. The spilled brandy crawled after it.

"I didn't mean to be so blunt," Dr. Kennedy said. "He's alive and doing quite well, considering what happened."

Mike held his breath during the details of the accident. "I find stubborn patients often do very well," he said. "Tom's a prime example of that."

The grandfather clock in the front hall chimed nine times. "I didn't think it was that late," Dr. Kennedy said. "I have an early day tomorrow."

"It's only seven-thirty in Toronto," Mike said. "I'd be in the middle of dinner with my wife."

"You must be tired from the trip. I suggest you get a good night's rest before you deal with Tom."

Mike stared into the fireplace. "I hadn't given any thought as to how I would approach him. With what you've told me, it's going to be even more difficult."

Dr. Kennedy stretched. "All I can do is wish you good luck." He stretched again. "I'll see you in the morning."

Mike lingered in the library, gazing into the fire until the flames became dying embers. Two drinks dispensed in rapid succession, he plucked a novel from the many shelves, one in the Sherlock Holmes detective series.

Sleep wouldn't come easy tonight. And it didn't. He rose at

six. On an impulse, he took a taxi to his brother's house, not at all sure what he would do once he arrived. As the car turned the corner, three men headed to the door and knocked. Dressed for outside work, he assumed they were longshoremen, Tom's co-workers.

"Stop here," Mike said to the driver, and watched the men take off their hats to greet the slender woman dressed in black who answered the door. Mike stared at her. Elegant was the word that sprang to mind. This must be Alice. He had come to know her through years of letters. She was more than words on paper now, and his heart throbbed with sorrow for her loss. The bags under her eyes, and reddened nose, indicated she had cried most of the night. Her face was grey, marked with grief, yet still revealed the pretty girl she must have been in her youth. A tall, handsome young man appeared behind her.

"Oh, my," Mike whispered.

"Are you all right, buddy?" the taxi man asked.

Mikes couldn't tear his eyes from Henry. "Yes. Yes," he said.

The young man resembled his own son, could have been an identical twin except for the hair colour. His youngest son was blond like his mother's family.

"Take me back," Mike said when the three men went inside.

"WE'RE SOME SORRY ABOUT YOUR mother, missus," Bill said. The other men mumbled agreement.

Alice smiled her thanks. "Would you like a cup of tea to warm up?"

Bill stood with his hat in hand. "No, thank you, missus," he said. "Me and the boys got together at work and took up a collection for you." He withdrew a large manila envelope from his coat pocket. "It should keep you going for a while."

Henry opened his mouth to speak.

Bill cut him off. "I know what you're going to say. We know you have some money saved up for medical school." He held up the envelope and continued. "The men agreed you need every penny you've saved for that. Son, times will be hard for your family, and you're out of work as well, with the Hull Home gone."

A dockworker next to Bill spoke to Alice. "Missus, it's not a handout. Tom dug deep into his pockets whenever one of us was laid up."

Alice accepted the envelope and laid it on the table. "I appreciate your generosity," she said. "So will Tom."

Bill turned to leave with the others and was partway out of the kitchen when he hesitated. "Missus, I'm some sorry I couldn't help Tom out on the ship."

"That's the third accident this month," Henry said. "The ones responsible for the equipment's safety are to blame, not you."

Alice sat at the table while Henry escorted the men out. She dried her eyes when he returned. "A fine bunch of men," she said. "Especially Bill. Mom really liked him." Alice sobbed into her hands. "If only she'd moved in here last night like we wanted."

Henry didn't know how to console her, or if anything could.

THE EVENING CLOSED IN ON St. John's. The stars flickered like crystal chips in a clear, black sky. People hurried home from work. Women cooked supper. Children played in the snow. The last autopsy concluded in the basement at the General Hospital. Thirty-four bodies. Some burned beyond recognition. Others without a single mark. They shared two common features. All perished at Hull Home. All died from smoke inhalation.

Dr. Kennedy stood next to the man who had signed every death certificate. Dr. Sharpe pulled the sheet over Dot's face. "This lady was in excellent health for her age." He sighed, his voice barely audible. "She didn't suffer, Frank. Maybe that'll bring some small comfort to the family."

Dr. Kennedy wheeled the body into the freezer. "God bless you, Dot," he whispered before shutting the heavy metal door on her. He took off the white hospital coat and hung it up. "The judicial inquiry into the fire begins the week after next. I'm not looking forward to that."

Dr. Sharpe scrubbed his hands. "I want to get my testimony over with as soon as possible." He looked at his colleague. "And to think Valentine's Day is just around the corner."

"A time to honour loved ones." Dr. Kennedy shook his head as if trying to shed himself of unwanted thoughts. "I heard Sir Edward Emerson will head the inquiry."

"That's right. He's a no-nonsense man who'll cut through the bull and get to the truth." Dr. Sharpe turned off the morgue light switch and shut the door. The two men walked down the long, dimly lit corridor. There was no one to hear the echo of their footsteps. They came to the elevator, slowed, looked at each other, then moved on to the stairs. Neither one wished to be confined to the limited space of the elevator. They parted on the main floor, Dr. Sharpe to his office, Dr. Kennedy to the parking lot.

Mrs. Simms had supper on the table when he arrived home. "Stew with dumplings and tea buns," she said. "Dr. Gibbs gave me a hand with the buns." She flushed a dark pink. "He's some handy in the kitchen."

Dr. Kennedy smiled despite the chill in his heart.

"All autopsies completed?" Mike asked when the housekeeper left to bring in dessert.

"I've witnessed plenty of terrible sights in my experience as a doctor. This was the worst."

"Frankie, do you think I should go home and forget about confronting Tom? He and Alice have enough to contend with."

"Alice needs some peace of mind more than ever right now." The doctor tore off a huge piece of bun. "So, no. You do what you came here to do."

Mrs. Simms brought in an apple crumble fresh from the oven and a second pot of tea. "There's another meeting about Confederation at seven," she said, cutting out two portions of the apple crumble. "I don't want to be late. The dishes can wait till I get back."

Dr. Kennedy looked at Mike. "I don't ever recall the woman asking my permission for anything," he said, as if she had already departed.

Mrs. Simms peered sideways at her employer. "Now, sir," she said. "You know darn well there's not a single word of truth in that."

"Confederation," Mike said. "I heard a radio interview with a Mr. Joseph Smallwood about that a week ago."

The housekeeper's expression became sullen. "He wants Newfoundland to become a Canadian province." She threw her hands up in the air. "I never heard the like before."

"There are many benefits to being Canadian," Mike said.

Mrs. Simms planted hands firmly on her wide hips. "And here I was thinking you were a fine fellow." A knock on the front door prevented further comment.

Dr. Kennedy helped himself to an extra serving of apple crumble. "I hope that's not an emergency call."

"I'm leaving now, so I'll send in whoever it is on my way out." Mrs. Simms left the room to get her coat and boots in the foyer.

Henry came into the dining room. His eyes went directly to Mike. "You look like Dad," he said.

Dr. Kennedy threw down his napkin. "Is your mother all right?" he said, rising from his chair.

"That's not why I'm here," Henry said. "With Dad's accident and Gran's death, Mom's forgotten about Uncle Mike. I had to see if he came."

"I didn't want to intrude on your grief just yet," Mike said. "And make matters worse."

"I agreed," Dr. Kennedy added. "It's better for your mother to wait until after Dot's funeral."

Henry nodded. "That's what I thought."

"Sit down," Dr. Kennedy said. "You're whiter than flour." He sweetened tea for Henry and made him drink at least half. "I didn't get to the hospital today. How's Mary?"

Henry held the cup between his hands. "She's still unconscious and hooked up to machines."

The doctor passed him a piece of apple crumble. "Mary's a strong girl. She'll pull through."

Henry stared into his cup. The tea shivered like water when a rock is skimmed along the surface.

Dr. Kennedy clapped a hand on his shoulder. "Don't give up on her."

Henry turned to Mike. "Why didn't you come home for your parents' funerals?" A nerve ticked in his jaw.

"You don't waste time in getting to the point." Mike smiled. "You father did the same even as a boy."

"Answer the question."

"When my father died," Mike said quietly, "I wrote my mother explaining why I couldn't get home."

"It goes without saying the excuse didn't satisfy Dad," Henry said.

"I send Tom a telegram when Mom died," Mike continued. "And tried for years to contact your father by letters, telegrams, phone calls."

Henry dragged a hand over his face. "What possible reason could justify not returning home for your parents' funerals?"

Mike pushed back his chair and stood up.

"Sweet Jesus!" Henry gasped.

Chapter 11

FIVE DAYS AFTER THE FIRE, many of the deceased residents from Hull Home were buried on a sunny morning in cemeteries all over the city, the choice of resting place dictated by the person's religion. Church bells tolled—a message to the living to reflect upon what had been taken away. The procession for Dot moved up Patrick Street to begin the final journey. The coffin rested on a sled drawn by a big, black horse. Its nostrils flared, the breath escaping like smoke out of a chimney. The animal climbed the hill and whinnied when it slid back a few paces on an ice patch. The driver calmed the horse and it began the task once again. Near the top the *clap-clap* of hooves was cushioned by layers of packed snow. Alice rode behind her mother, silent, dry-eyed, gloved hands on her lap. Cars along the route stopped in respect and waited for the hearse to pass, as did people in the street. The aftertaste of death permeated the city.

The horse turned in to the gate of Mount Carmel Cemetery, the graveyard for Roman Catholics, which overlooked Quidi Vidi Lake. Dot was laid to rest alongside her husband, who had passed nearly three decades earlier, a casualty of the Spanish flu pandemic of 1918. Tom had insisted on attending and had released himself from the hospital. He sat between Alice and Henry, their heads bowed for Dot's last blessing.

The priest made the sign of the Cross over the coffin. "Rest in peace, dear friend," he murmured, blinking away a tear from the corner of his eye. "We'll see each other again, God willing."

"Thank you, Father Whitten," Alice said. "Mom would be some delighted if she knew her oldest friend in the world presided over her funeral."

"Dot wouldn't stand for anything less," he said, a quiver in his voice. "Nothing will ever be the same without her." He glanced at the coffin. "My last conversation with her was the night before the fire at the Home. She told me how excited she was about the vote on Confederation."

"If I knew Dot," Tom said, "I'd say she was all for it."

"Indeed she was. And determined to win you over."

Tom nodded. "If anyone could, it was her."

"I must say my farewell," Father Whitten said. "Mr. Duggan asked me to do his wife's service."

"His dog, Rusty, is the only thing keeping him going," Alice said. "It's sad they weren't blessed with children."

The priest smiled at Henry. "Dot spoke often of you. The doctor-to-be, she'd say. Needless to say your grandmother was delighted beyond words about that."

"I miss her," Henry said. "She was easy to talk to."

"And gave her opinion whether you liked it or not." The priest smiled to himself. "A great lady. Before I go, Alice, promise me you'll keep in touch."

"Well, now, Father, you married my parents and me, you baptized me and Henry, and you've attended every special occasion in my life." She hugged the retired priest. "Mom would never forgive me if I didn't."

"Here's my ride," Father Whitten said as a young priest from St. Patrick's Church drove toward them. "I'll call you tomorrow." Alice watched him walk away, his step less lively than the last time she saw him.

Bill made his way through the crowd. "I'm some sorry, missus," he said. "Mrs. Gatherall was a lovely lady."

Alice smiled, but it didn't reach her eyes. "Thank you, Bill."

Well-wishers and mourners expressed their condolences one by one as they filed past.

The cemetery all but deserted, Alice kissed the brass-rimmed coffin. "Dad's waited a long time for you, Mom. Be happy."

Henry and Bill helped Tom to the car. "You haven't missed much work," Bill said. "What with icebergs and packed ice, everything is slowed to a standstill."

"I'm going to walk home," Henry said.

"That'll take at least an hour," Alice said. "You'll freeze."

Tom snuggled close to his wife. "Alice, love," he said softly, putting an arm around her. "Our son isn't a baby anymore." He turned to Henry. "We'll have piping hot tea waiting when you get home."

"Thanks, Dad." Henry shut the door and moved down the footpath between the long rows of headstones which lead to the rear entrance, a shortcut to the boulevard. Dr. Kennedy's car honked at him on the way down Kennas Hill. He pulled a hand from his pocket to wave to his parents. Something dropped to the ground.

He picked up the ticket stub from Silver's Jewellery Store. The snow caked his fingertips and stung like needle pricks.

"Oh, Gran, I forgot all about the locket." He turned left toward downtown, keeping to one side of the street to avoid contact with the charred remains of Hull Home, and hopped on the streetcar. Someone touched his shoulder from the seat behind. He turned, sneaking a quick glance at the skeleton that had been his place of work and his grandmother's home. "Hello, Dougie."

The boy sat with one hand in his pocket, his head to the side, his face grey. "I'm on my way to buy Mary a box of candy for Valentine's Day," he said. "Mom says they'll help her come back to us when she feels how much we care." Dougie's eyes glossed over. "Henry, do you believe that's true?"

"Yes, I do."

Dougie opened his hand to reveal a hard candy made from boiled molasses and brown sugar. "You know how much Mary loves Bullseyes."

"She sure does," Henry said.

The streetcar jolted to a stop. "I get off here," Dougie said. "See ya." His arms dangled like rubber tubes.

Henry disembarked at the next stop. The clerk looked up from paperwork when the bell over the door jangled. Wire-rimmed glasses hovered off the end of his nose. "I see your grandmother isn't with you today," he said.

"Gran died in the fire."

The clerk readjusted his glasses. "I am terribly sorry. Please forgive my insensitivity."

"You had no way of knowing."

The clerk took the ticket stub and pulled out a drawer from a side cabinet. He withdrew a small box wrapped in white tissue with a red ribbon. "Here you are," he said. "I hope it brings some small comfort to your mother."

“Me, too,” Henry said. He wondered if the locket would be a bitter reminder that Dot was gone forever.

The temperature seemed to be stuck well below zero since the beginning of winter. Yet Henry was oblivious to the weather, to the passersby, even to the smell from the bakery that, without fail, used to conjure up images of Mary and laughter and happy times spent with his grandmother. Henry felt weary and knew it had nothing to do with physical exertion. He neared his house. The walls would suffocate him. Before he realized it, St. Clare’s Hospital rose up before him, big, grey, sterile.

Henry scaled the stairs to the third floor.

“Miss Norris’s condition hasn’t changed,” the nurse at the station said to his inquiry.

His weariness intensified. “Can I see her?”

“Visiting hours are not till this afternoon.”

Henry ran a hand over his eyes.

The nurse smiled. “Seeing as she’s in a private room, you won’t disturb any other patients. Go ahead.”

Henry opened the door, hesitant to go in. This was the first time he had seen her since the day of the fire. Rather, the first time he’d had the nerve to face her. The splotches of blood and soot cleaned away, she looked beautiful, peaceful.

He moved a chair closer to the bed. “Mary, you probably don’t want me to be here. Who can blame you?” He touched her cheek. She felt warm, soft. “Please give me the chance to explain, to apologize.”

Henry leaned on the bed rail and stared down at Mary. He watched her chest rise and fall in a steady, even pattern. The sun travelled around the room, shifting, changing shadows. He didn’t stir. Neither did Mary. His heart ached. The clatter of meal trays in the corridor broke his concentration. "I have to go, Mary. Goodbye for now."

Henry passed acquaintances on the way home. All took the time to extend their sincere sorrow. *Thank you* became ingrained in his brain, uttered without thought like a child reciting a memorized poem in front of his classmates. Snow began to fall, light at first, then maddened into a whipping assault. Henry bent his head into his chest and ran. He reached his house and barrelled inside to rid himself of the clinging snow and the . . . if only he could verbalize the array of emotions tearing at him, each one in a battle to overthrow the other.

"Where were you?" Alice asked. "I was worried."

Henry stood by the stove to thaw out. His numb cheeks prickled when the heat frolicked around his face. "I went to see Mary." He pulled the gift box out of his pocket. "First I picked this up at Silver's Jewellery."

"I'd forgotten tomorrow is Valentine's Day," Alice said. "Mary will love whatever you bought for her."

"It's not for Mary. This is the reason Gran asked me to take her shopping last week."

"Dear Mom. She wanted to surprise me."

"She said that fifty is a milestone and had to be celebrated with a special present."

Henry held out the box to his mother. "Even though your birthday's not till tomorrow, Gran wouldn't mind you having it a day early."

Alice untied the ribbon and unwrapped the paper like they were precious, delicate items made by Dot herself. The silver heart shone on white satin. "It's lovely."

"Gran had it engraved," Henry said.

Alice clicked the locket cover open. "'Alice, my joy,'" she

read. "'You make me proud.'" She clasped the silver heart to her chest. "Oh, Henry. You'll never know what this message means to me."

"I was afraid it might make you sadder."

Alice threw her arms around Henry. "The locket is a perfect keepsake from Mom. I'll keep it always."

Tom, concealed from sight, turned away from the side of the kitchen door and took a deep breath to quash the rising lump in his throat. "Thank you, Dot," he whispered. "Alice needed that. So did I." He hobbled down the hall to the living room using his crutches and fell into an armchair. He dragged each foot onto a small, cushioned stool. His heels hung over the edge.

A light rap on the front door was followed by a blast of cold air with Dr. Kennedy in its wake. "I came by to see how you're doing," he said. "Since you left the hospital without specific instructions about your care."

Tom rubbed the crease between his brows. "How long before I can go back to work is all I need to know."

"Several months."

Tom almost came out of the chair. "Tell me that's a joke."

"Tom, the bones in your heels weren't just broken, they were crushed. Do as I say to make sure they heal properly. Or would you prefer to walk with canes for the rest of your life?" The doctor moved the crutches out of Tom's reach. "You only use these to come downstairs in the morning, go to the toilet, and back upstairs at night."

"For how long?"

"Until I say otherwise." Dr. Kennedy glared at Tom. "You understand me?"

"All right. I don't have to like it, though."

"You don't have to sook like a youngster either."

Tom looked toward the window next to the fireplace. "The damn icicles are back," he said to himself.

"What was that?"

"Nothing important," Tom said.

There was a knock on the door.

Alice entered the room with Henry and Fred Russell. She held three bags of crinkles. "A little something for you and the missus," Fred said. "I know how much you all love our crinkles."

"How about a nice cup of tea and a crinkle for everyone?" Alice said.

"Lovely, Mrs. Gibbs," Fred said. "At a time like this it must've been some good to meet your brother-in-law after all these years."

"What?" Tom said, his body rigid.

Alice and Henry exchanged a look.

Tom sat up straight. "What's he talking about?"

"I was in the back when he came into the bakery. He hasn't changed much. The scattered grey hair and wrinkle is all."

Tom looked at his wife. "Did you know about this?" An icicle dropped and plunked onto the window ledge.

Alice stared at him like a child stranded among strangers, hoping to see a familiar face. "Tom, you . . . you know I never go to the bakery."

Tom's eyes slithered to his son. "What about you?"

Fred flushed. "I'm real sorry, folks. Didn't mean to start a ruckus." He slapped on his hat. "I'd best get back to work," he said, and scurried out of the living room.

"Take it easy, Tom," Dr. Kennedy said. "I mentioned Mike to them on the phone before I came over. He's here as a favour to me. A medical consultation concerning one of my patients."

Alice knelt beside her husband. "Tom, this is a good opportunity for you to talk to him, to have all your questions answered."

"I don't have any questions where he's concerned."

"Tom, please."

"Alice, normally I'd do anything for you."

She got up and moved a few feet from Tom. "I see. This is the one thing you can't . . . or should I say, the one thing you won't do for me."

"I'm sorry, love. If Mike has the gall to come to the house, don't let him in. I have nothing to say to my brother." A second icicle cracked off. Dr. Kennedy picked up his medical bag from the coffee table. "Tom, I never thought you were this selfish." He gave Henry a glance and, with a tilt of his head, signalled him to go down the hall. Henry followed him into the porch.

"Thanks for the help in there," Henry said. "That was a close call."

Dr. Kennedy picked up his coat from the bannister. "You're well aware Mike's determined to have it out with Tom. Maybe you should warn your mother that he's decided to do it tomorrow night."

Alice came out from the living room. "You think on your feet, Doctor," she said, "which I really do appreciate."

"Anytime, Alice," he said, buttoning his coat.

"I don't know what to make of Tom. He becomes a stranger at the mere mention of Mike."

"Not a stranger," the doctor said. "A spoiled brat who demands his own way is more like it." He half grinned. "If you don't mind me saying so, that is."

"Like my father used to be fond of saying," Alice said. "The truth at all costs."

"Mom." Henry lowered his voice. "Mike's coming by tomorrow night."

"Perhaps it's just as well," Alice said. "I want to get it over with."

"I can come over for moral support," Dr. Kennedy said.

Alice brightened somewhat. "The coward in me is happy to accept your offer," she said, and went to the kitchen.

The doctor put on his gloves. "Henry, make sure Tom stays off his feet as much as possible."

A LOUD CRASH AND A squeal from the kitchen devoured the doctor's last words.

"Mom," Henry cried out, and flew down the hall.

Tom attempted to stand and toppled over. "Alice, are you all right?" he yelled, pulling himself into a sitting position.

"Stay where you are, Tom," Dr. Kennedy said before hurrying after Henry.

Alice lay sprawled on her back, fragments of broken plates scattered around her. Henry bent down to help her up.

"Don't touch her," the doctor ordered. He checked her back with practised precision. "Nothing broken," he said.

"I was getting dishes down from the cupboard and didn't see the water on the floor," Alice said.

"What's going on?" Tom called.

Henry helped his mother to a chair. "Don't make a fuss over nothing at all," she said.

Tom crawled into the kitchen and gaped at the mess on the floor. "Alice, are you hurt?"

"Embarrassed is more like it. I was a bit clumsy."

Dr. Kennedy took her pulse. "You've had a hard time lately, with Dot's passing and your husband's accident." He gave Tom a severe look. “It’s a wonder your wife is not huddling in bed under the covers with all the stress she’s under.”

ALICE LOOKED AT THE CLOCK on the night table. Three in the morning. She had slept for an hour. Thirty minutes more than the night before. The house was colder than Dot’s homemade ice cream. She slipped out of bed and tiptoed into the hallway. Henry’s door was open. He flung his arm over the side of the bed, throwing the covers down to his waist. About to move on, she heard him utter a name: “Mary.” Alice walked quietly to her son and pulled the blankets over his shoulders. “I’m sorry, Henry. Life isn’t always fair.”

Henry moaned softly. Alice moved back into the hall, making for her mother’s room at the front of the house. The scent of lilacs, Dot’s favourite perfume, washed over her as she sat in the rocking chair her father had made when she was a little girl. “How do I live without you, Mom?” The *creak, creak* of the chair disturbed the silence. “I was depending on you to help with Mike and Tom.”

A car chugged to a stop outside the window. Alice looked to see who was about so early in the morning. Flora Norris and Dougie hurried from their house into a taxi. “Please, God, not Mary, too,” Alice cried into the quiet, sleeping house.

Chapter 12

ALICE SHOOK HER SON, ALMOST hauling him from the bed. "Henry, wake up. You have to go to St. Clare's right away."

Henry bolted upright. "What's wrong?" he said, his voice groggy. His mother's face was a blur among shadows in the dim light.

Alice tugged on his arm. "Get out of bed."

"Is Dad all right?"

Alice pulled the quilts down. "Your father's asleep. Hurry up and get dressed."

Henry's heart pounded against his ribs. "I don't understand," he said, shivering, his toes bunched up on the cold floor. "Are you sick?"

Alice pushed him toward the closet. "Flora and Dougie are on their way to the hospital. I saw them from the window. There's nowhere else they'd be going this hour in the morning."

Henry faltered a step and reached out for the wall to support him, a dazed expression on his face.

"Get a move on," Alice said. "I'll call you a taxi."

Henry hauled on his trousers. "No. I'd walk there before

the taxi got here." He pulled a sweater over his head and shot past his mother down the stairs.

Henry shoved his foot into a boot, hopping on the other one until he lost his balance and teetered. He sat on the hall chair to put on the other one.

"Don't forget to let me know as soon as you hear anything," Alice said.

Henry's coat, wide open, flapped in the wind. The tails whipped behind him as he raced down the road like a starved wolf on the scent of food. He wore neither hat nor gloves. His thoughts centred on Mary. What if she was dead? No, he shouldn't waste good energy on what-if. Gran wouldn't approve of that. To keep his mind vacant, he counted the crunch of his footsteps.

One, two, three, four. His heart pumped at the same pace. Five, six, seven, eight. Longer strides. Nine, ten, eleven. Running. His heart galloped even faster. The moon kept pace with Henry, the orb's face animated. Laughing? Crying? The answer depended on the person who gazed up.

Henry started for the hospital's main entrance and travelled several yards, when he stopped abruptly. "Damn it," he grumbled, remembering the emergency entrance was the only door open after hours. He retraced his steps back to LeMarchant Road. Five people sat in the waiting room. A boy about seventeen with a handkerchief to a gash over his eye was called into an examination room as Henry hurried down the hall to the stairs.

Stop, the moon seemed to say when Henry reached the door to Mary's floor. He stared out the side window at the white ball. *What if she's dead?* it taunted. *You don't deserve to see her.*

Henry gripped the door handle. Why didn't he have the strength to pull the door open?

"Are you all right?"

Henry gawked at a nurse.

"You're the young man I let see Miss Morris before visiting hours began."

"H . . . how is she? I know Mrs. Norris was called here a little while ago."

"I can only give out that information to family," Nurse Franklin said. She opened the door. "Wait at the nurses' station and I'll tell Mrs. Norris you'd like to see her." She walked down the hall, her white shoes squishing softly on the newly waxed floor.

Henry stared after her. A pulse pounded in his ears, his palms so sweaty that water dripped down his fingers. The young nurse behind the desk looked up from her paperwork to give him a reassuring smile. Henry looked down the hall once more. Nurse Franklin reached Mary's door and disappeared inside.

Flora turned to the nurse. The heavy circles under her eyes blended in with the dark shadows, giving her face a mask-like appearance. She held Mary's hand. Dougie sat opposite his mother, his arms flung over the side of the bed, his head nestled between them. The candy he had bought for his sister sat unopened in a red box on the nightstand. "I don't want to leave her yet," Flora said.

"That's not a problem," Nurse Franklin said. "There's a young man here asking about your daughter. What would you like me to tell him?"

"Please tell him I'll be out in a second," Flora said. She gently released her daughter's hand.

"Mom." Mary's eyelids flickered open, her eyes heavy and

unfocused. She stared through the haze of a long, deep sleep. "Where are you going?"

Flora leaned in close to the bed. "Don't worry, love. Henry's here. I'll just have a quick word with him and be right back."

Mary coughed. A sound like the scraping of a rusty barrel. She grabbed at her chest, her face contorted in pain.

Dougie looked at his mother with big round eyes.

"I'm all right," Mary said. "I ache a smidgen, that's all."

"Dougie," Flora said. "Go tell Henry I'll be a minute or so. You wait with him."

Dougie hesitated. "Mary, are you really all right?"

She smiled as best she could. "Would I lie to you?"

A broad smile lit up his face. "Henry will be some happy you're awake," he said, and hurried away.

Mary rubbed the side of her head.

"I can have the nurse give you something for the pain," Flora said.

"Nothing works." Tears spilled down the sides of Mary's face to the pillow. "Mom, I'm sorry to put you through this."

Flora smoothed hair away from her daughter's bruised cheek. "My sweet girl," she said softly. "This isn't your fault. Does Henry know?"

Mary turned her head to the wall. "I don't want him to."

"You should tell him."

"Oh, Mom. Don't you see? That's the last thing I want. Especially now he's going away."

"Don't cry, love. We'll figure out something."

Mary sniffed. "It's too late for that."

Flora sighed. It sounded more like a shudder.

"Mom, I want to tell Dougie in my own time. He's had enough to deal with."

"I'll tell Henry you're awake and send him away."

"No. I want to see him."

Flora kissed her daughter's forehead. "Are you sure you're up to it?"

"Yes."

MARY FORCED HER EYES OPEN when Henry called her name. He stood over the bed. The stubble on his face made him look older, tired, defeated. "Why are you here?" she asked.

"Mom saw your mother and Dougie leave the house. We thought . . ." He gulped, not able to finish the sentence.

"Mom asked the hospital to call as soon as I woke up."

Henry sat in Dougie's chair. The urge to take Mary in his arms and simply hold her made him tremble. "Mom and Dad will be beside themselves when they hear you're awake and on the mend."

"Henry, I'm real sorry about your grandmother. She wouldn't leave until all the residents were out." Mary shuddered. "Honest to God, she didn't suffer. The smoke got to her before the roof fell in on us."

"The doctor in charge of autopsies told us." Henry moved his chair closer to the bed. "Mary, when you're well enough, we have to talk."

She coughed, a soft throat tickle at first, then it grew into a steady hacking that tensed every muscle in her body and choked off her breath. Sweat drenched her face as she struggled to take in air, her face redder than a fresh sunburn.

Henry jumped to his feet. "I'll get the nurse."

Mary stilled him with the touch of her hand on his arm. "No," she whispered. "I have something to say to you."

"It can wait until you're home."

"We aren't going out together anymore, Henry. There's nothing left to talk about."

"Mary, please."

"My life will go on just fine without you. Be a doctor with my blessing." The words were laced with an edge Henry couldn't define. "I really do wish you all the best." She closed her eyes. "I'm tired. Please ask Mom and Dougie to come back in."

ALICE SAT IN THE LIVING room wrapped in a blue-and-red checkered quilt. Four in the morning and still no word from Henry. Her mind invoked the worst images, so she threw off the quilt and lit the hall and kitchen stoves. She returned to the armchair and looked out the window at the empty street. A scattering of snowflakes floated down. Her eyes fastened on a large one and she watched its descent to the sidewalk. She looked up to see Henry walk toward the house. His head low, his collar turned up, his face was a hidden mystery.

Alice said a silent prayer.

"Mary's awake," Henry said as soon as he came through the door. "I was going to telephone but didn't want to wake Dad."

Alice took his coat, shook off the snow, and hung it up. "I'll put the kettle on," she said, and set about making toast for both of them.

Henry drank the steaming liquid, savouring the warmth as it slid down his throat. "Mary's coming along, considering all her injuries," he said. "She'll be in hospital for at least another week."

"I was in a state the whole time you were gone," Alice said. "It's like a gift from heaven to hear a piece of happy news." She put extra Carnation milk into her tea. "Did you get a chance to see Mary?"

"She gave me her blessing to go away."

"That bothers you?"

The wind howled, rattling in the chimney, slamming into the house. Henry banged his cup down on the table. Tea slopped onto his hand, scalding the skin. "Will this goddamned winter ever end?"

"Your grandmother would have a witty reply to that," Alice said softly.

The thump of crutches on the floor heralded Tom's entrance into the kitchen. He wore rumpled long johns and his hair was in disarray. "There you are," he said. "When I woke up and found the two of you gone, I had the fright of my life. What are you doing up this early anyway?"

Alice related the circumstances. "It's going on five," she said at the conclusion of the story. "I might as well get dressed and start breakfast."

"Henry," Tom said when his wife left, "what's on your mind?"

Henry looked at his father but said nothing.

Tom pulled his chair closer to the table, making it hop like a jackrabbit. "I'm well aware that things have been strained between us lately. A fool could see you're twisting in the wind about something which has nothing to do with that issue between us." He looked at Henry with kind eyes. "That doesn't change the fact that you're still my son."

"Mary believes my applying for medical school proves I never really cared for her." He shook his head as if the words ate at his very core. "She says I used her."

"Only you know the truth on that score, son."

Henry glanced out the window to conceal his surprise to his father's response. The light snow had become a steady downfall. "I've given it a lot of thought the last few days, Dad. Maybe Mary has a point."

"Which is?" Tom said softly.

"I didn't realize how much she meant to me until the fire. She deserves better than I gave her."

"The way I see it," Tom said, "words are about as cheap as horseshit lying about on the street when feelings are involved." He sat back. "Show Mary what you think of her. That way she'll see right into your heart."

"That sounds like the kind of advice Gran would give," Henry said. "I still can't believe she's gone."

Tom smiled. "Who do you think taught me how to be so wise?" The sparkle left his eyes. "Dot was one fine lady who should still be with us." Static replaced the music on the radio.

Tom glared at the brown box. "Turn that damn nuisance off."

Henry obliged without hesitation. "Mary said Gran tried to save as many residents as possible."

Tom balled his hands into fists. "It's Hull's fault your grandmother's dead." He breathed deeply to calm down. "I heard the stove caused the fire. How often did Mary tell us Hull tried to fix it himself instead of getting a proper mechanic in?"

"Mr. Freeman did warn him often enough about that," Henry said.

"If there's any justice in this world, he should be charged with manslaughter."

Alice put the *Daily News* on the kitchen counter. "Dougie's a lot more chipper this morning," she said with a smile, glancing at the front-page headline. Her smile vanished.

"What's the matter, Mom?" Henry said.

"The hearing for the fire begins the twenty-first. I didn't expect it to be so soon."

"The hearing will be tough," Tom said. "We'll get through it as a family."

Alice sat in Dot's place at the table. She smoothed down the cloth placemat her mother had made a few months earlier. "It's difficult to imagine that I'll never see my mother again."

Chapter 13

THE TEMPERATURE HAD REMAINED AT fifteen below zero during the day, dipping another ten degrees by suppertime. The wind swirled around the house, groping, searching for a way inside. Icicles hung like shark's teeth, sharp and uneven from every window. They peered in at Tom, boasting their prowess, taunting him. He looked toward his crutches and felt a spasm of helplessness. His efforts to get rid of them had only made them more aggressive, intent on returning stronger and bigger than before.

Tom tore his eyes from the window and buried his head in the *Evening Telegram*. Bright yellow-orange flames popped and hissed in the grate. Thanks to the hall stove and the fireplace, the living room was warm, inviting. Alice darned the heel of her husband's woollen work sock. Three more pairs lay on the couch beside her waiting their turn. Every now and again she would pause and stare into the fire.

Henry's head hung over a Sherlock Holmes novel. He had read the same paragraph three times and couldn't recall a word. The grandfather clock in the corner chimed eight times. Henry glanced at his mother. She sat tall, her hands still, looking at the clock as if counting the chimes. He felt her anxiety, thick in the air, seep into him. It'll be all right, he wished he could tell her, and went back to the book and the same paragraph.

"Ow!" Alice yelped. A drop of blood landed on her dress. Henry and Tom looked at her. "I pricked my finger," she said, sucking the tip of her thumb.

"That's a first," Tom said. "You can darn socks in the dark without a hitch. Love, time will lessen the heartache of Dot's loss."

Henry caught his mother's eyes. If Dad only knew the real reason for her nerves, he thought. Her expression seemed to question why Mike was not here. She turned to her husband, who had gone back to the paper.

"Smallwood's made the headlines again," Tom said. "He's like a spider after a fly when it comes to Confederation."

"What does he have to say this time?" Alice asked. Henry sensed a hint of anxiety which he knew had little to do with Confederation.

"The man's still flapping his gums about all the wonderful benefits we'll receive as Canadians." Tom bunched up the *Telegram* and threw it into the fire. "Makes you wonder what he's getting out of it."

He wants the best for Newfoundland, Henry nearly said out loud.

All three watched the paper shrivel and crumble into ashes.

Tom pointed to the black soot. "That's what will happen to Newfoundland if Smallwood gets his way."

"Dad, change can be good."

Tom continued to gaze into the fire. "None that I've lived through," he said so quietly Henry wasn't sure he heard him correctly. The crackle in the grate competed with the rumble of the wind in the chimney.

Three raps sounded on the door. Alice dropped the darning on her lap. The needle slid down her leg, dangling close to the floor like a hanged man. "Oh, my," she cried out.

Tom roused himself from his reverie. "Goodness, love, it's only someone at the front door."

Alice gathered up her work. "I reckon Dr. Kennedy's right," she said. "My nerves are stretched to the breaking point."

A second round of louder knocks blasted into the room. "I'll get that," Henry said, forcing his voice to sound calm. Through the glass at the top of the door he saw the shape of a man. Mike. The spectre of many long-ago Christmases. Would his father allow himself to face this ghost?

Mike's hands were deep in his pockets. A scarf covered his neck and ears. "I don't ever remember it being this cold," he said.

"Neither does anyone else."

"Who is it?" Tom called.

Mike leaned a hand against the wall for support and wiped his feet on the hall mat. He gave his nephew a look which said it's now or never and walked to the living room with an almost undetectable limp. "It's me, Tommy," he said.

Tom's mouth moved, but no words came out.

Mike looked at Alice, a soft smile on his face. "Hello, sister-in-law. It's wonderful to finally meet you."

"It's incredible," Alice said. "You're a perfect, older version of Tom."

Mike chuckled. "I've been told worse things."

"I don't want you in my home," Tom spat out. "Leave now."

"Alice, Henry, I'd like to speak with my brother in private, if you don't mind."

“I mind,” Tom snapped.

“We’ll be in the kitchen,” Alice said, and fled from the room with Henry.

Tom gripped the arms of his chair. “I have nothing to say to you. Get out.”

Mike stepped forward. “Well, I have much to say to you.” He advanced farther into the room. “The least you can do is listen. You owe me that much.”

Tom laughed, a deep, guttural noise that conveyed no joy. “I owe you. What a joke.” He grabbed his crutches from the side of the armchair and tried to stand up. His heels slid from the stool, striking the floor with a thud. Tom winced in pain and flopped back into the chair.

“Frankie told me about your accident,” Mike said. “You’re lucky to be alive.”

Tom stared at the icicles outside the window, his face harder, colder.

Mike sat down on the couch. “You don’t know how difficult it was to leave our parents and you, Tommy, a ten-year-old boy who believed I could do no wrong.”

“I outgrew that years ago.” Tom kept his eyes fixed on the icicles.

“My loneliness was like a sore that wouldn’t heal. My new life wasn’t easy, Tommy.”

“Don’t call me that,” Tom said. “I’m not a child anymore.”

“Not being able to get home for Mom or Dad’s funeral tore me apart. I had no choice in the matter.”

Tom’s face reddened. Even his ears glowed. “Tore you apart.” His voice quivered. “Had no choice. Do you truly believe you’re talking to the gullible youngster who used to hang on your every word?” The veins in his neck bulged out like thick rope. “You have some gall. This is the last time I will tell you to get out of my house.”

Mike got to his feet slowly. “I’ll go for now. However, you’re not the only one with a stubborn streak. You will hear me out one way or another.”

Alice came back into the living room when she heard the front door close. Tom looked into the fireplace. She looked at her husband’s profile. A sinew in his jaw ticked like a rapid heartbeat. “What did Mike have to say for himself?” she said.

Tom turned to her, his face white. “Where’s Henry?”

“Don’t try to change the subject, Tom Gibbs. This is important.”

“I’m beat, Alice. Besides, it’s time for bed.” He muttered and grumbled at his sore arm muscles as he pushed himself up. “I want to go to bed. Where’s Henry?”

“Here,” Henry said, hurrying from the kitchen. “Are you all right?”

“I want to go upstairs.”

Henry passed the crutches to his father and followed him up the stairs, a buffer in case he tumbled backwards. Tom didn’t utter a word, bringing down the tips of the wooden sticks on every step a little harder than was necessary. He stayed silent while Alice helped him undress.

“He still has his Newfoundland accent,” she said when they were in bed.

“What?”

“Mike . . . he still has it. You can’t take Newfoundland out of the person.”

“You can take him out of Newfoundland.”

Alice sighed inwardly. “How did you feel when you saw Mike?”

"Angry."

"Is that all?"

Tom looked sideways at his wife. "What would you like me to say?"

"The truth. Somewhere inside you must want to know what kept Mike away."

He was silent for a moment. "Dot wasn't a blood relative, but you know I thought the world of her."

Alice nuzzled closer to Tom. "She loved you, too. What does my mother have to do with Mike?"

"Distance wouldn't have prevented me from attending her funeral."

Alice smeared a tear across her cheek. "The little boy never really dies in a man," she said. "He's the one that must've been thrilled to see his little brother."

Tom's body became rigid. "You're wrong, Alice. Mike killed that child when he didn't show up the day our father was buried."

Alice looked up at her husband. His jaw locked tight, he stared out the window. Icicles stared back. "That's the hurt talking," she said, and turned off the lamp. "It's never too late to make amends."

DR. KENNEDY WAITED IN THE study for Mike's return. He cradled a whisky in one hand while browsing through a medical journal on tuberculosis.

The housekeeper looked in through the open door. "I'm off to bed," she said. "Is there anything I can get you before I go?"

"No, thank you, Mrs. Simms. Good night."

"I baked cheese buns in case you crave a little something to eat later on. They're cooling on the kitchen sink. Dr. Gibbs sure is partial to my buns." She giggled. "Good night, Doctor."

Dr. Kennedy chucked the journal aside. He glanced at the telephone on his desk, tempted to call the Gibbs house. "Don't be an idiot. What excuse will you give for calling at this late hour?"

"Ah," Mike said. "I see you still converse with yourself."

"Maybe if you didn't sneak up on people you wouldn't hear their private thoughts."

Mike looked at the drink cupped in his friend's hands. "I could use one of those," he said, and filled a glass to the rim.

"I take it the visit wasn't a success," the doctor said.

Mike gulped down the whisky. His hair was windblown, his nose red, his eyes watery from the cold. "You could say that." He poured a second drink. "Tommy . . . Tom didn't give me a chance to even begin an explanation."

Dr. Kennedy topped up his own glass. "Can't say as I blame him."

Mike sat down and looked at his friend. "Why would you say that?"

"Tom pined after you for years. He was a few years younger than Henry when your parents died within months of each other. He drew into himself, enlisted in the army, and went off to war." He took another swig of alcohol. "The boy came back bewildered, lonely—that is, until he met Alice. She brought purpose and love back into his life."

"How did they meet?"

"In my office. Alice left her gloves in the reception area. Tom, ever the chivalrous young man, chased her down the road to return them." Dr. Kennedy smiled. "Alice denies it, of course, but I'm sure she deliberately left the gloves behind."

Mike ran a finger around the rim of his glass. "She's a lovely woman."

"Tom's a fine man most days. What's your next step?"

“Keep at Tom until he listens.”

“Mike, why on earth didn’t you simply show him up front why you missed your parents’ funerals?”

“I wanted him to hear me out first. Why does my brother have to so inflexible?”

“Tom can be obstinate. Look at your own father.”

“True,” Mike said. “Once he latched onto something, it stuck tighter than a nail hammered in wood.” Mike ground a fist into his hand.

“You can’t be all that shocked about Tom’s reaction tonight. Why are you so upset about it?”

Mike went to the fireplace and looked into the dying embers. “For nearly forty years I kept Tommy alive in my heart. Tonight, reality smacked me in the face.” He turned to Dr. Kennedy. “Tommy’s gone, replaced with the man named Tom, who doesn’t want me back in his life.”

EARLY THE NEXT MORNING, HENRY woke to find the door he had left open the night before closed. Once awake, he could never stay in bed.

Tom Gibbs was sitting at the kitchen table with tea and toast when Henry strolled into the heated kitchen. “I lit the stoves this morning. A nice break for your mother.” He wore a housecoat and hadn’t shaved.

“I didn’t hear you pass my room,” Henry said.

Tom rubbed his two knees. “I crawled down the hall, shut your door so as not to disturb you, and came down the stairs on my backside.” He frowned. “It was a chore to drag the crutches along without making noise.”

Henry put bread on the toaster doors. “Dad, you don’t look like you closed your eyes the whole night.”

"Too much on my mind. What are you doing up so early?" A light grey smoke drifted up from the toaster. Tom made a face. "Don't know how you can eat burned bread."

Henry spread blueberry jam on the charred toast. "It tastes better that way." He licked his fingers. "It's time I look for a new job."

"Why?" Tom brushed invisible bread crumbs from his lap.

"You're laid up with no income, Dad. The money the longshoremen collected won't last forever. A few months' earnings will help tide us over until you get on your feet again."

"Any prospects lined up?"

Henry drank a little tea. "I spoke with Fred. The bakery doesn't need anyone."

"Maybe one of the downtown stores might need someone good with figures."

"I've made the rounds there." Henry chewed the crusty toast. "They don't want to take on someone who'll only be around a short while."

"Sounds reasonable."

"Bill says he'll put in a word for me at the dock."

Tom's lower lip twitched. "Good old Bill should mind his own business."

"He was against the idea, but I insisted. Besides, it'll only be temporary."

Tom pushed his plate away and leaned across the table, almost reaching his son. "Listen here, Henry. No one was happier than me when you didn't show any interest in the docks. Unloading cargo ships is godawful hard, not to mention dangerous work."

"But Dad—"

"Listen, Henry. Accidents happen on a weekly basis. Look

at me." He stared down at his feet. "I'd be dead if it wasn't for my war training. It's no place for a man with an education or one who has a grain of sense."

"Dad, you finished high school. Not too many of your generation accomplished that. Yet you gave up an office job at the butter factory for the docks."

"A move I've regretted ever since."

"Then why did you leave?"

"Your mother asked me that same question after we were married." Tom became quiet, mulling the answer over in his mind. "I was young, just back from a horrible war . . . and I was alone. All my buddies worked at the docks. I reckon I needed to be with them."

You still miss your brother, Henry thought. And you're too proud to admit it or to forgive him.

Tom handed his cup to Henry for a refill. "If I'd met your mother earlier," he said, "she would've knocked some sense into me." Tom stared at his son. "You'll be gone in a couple of months, won't you?"

Chapter 14

DOUGIE SKIPPED THE SHORT DISTANCE from the sidewalk to the Gibbs house, the first stop on his delivery route with the *Daily News*. He whistled "All Around the Circle," his head bobbing to the tune. Snow fell as it had all during the night. The white flakes covered his dark lashes and the blond hair poking out from the wool cap knitted by Dot a month earlier. His footprints had become faint indentations, soon to be obliterated. He rolled up the newspaper and was about to shove it through the mail slot when the door opened.

"Thought I heard you," Henry said. "Right on time, too."

"I have to be." Dougie passed over the paper. "Mom would kill me if I was late for school."

Henry looked down at his slippers, the toes covered in snow, and stepped back. He turned his eyes to the banks crowding the sidewalk. "I don't know where they're going to put all this new white stuff."

"Dump it into the harbour, I suppose," Dougie said in a singsong voice. Snow gathered on the bag slung across his chest.

"What are you so chipper about this early in the day?"

Dougie stuck out his tongue and caught a flake. "Mary's coming home today. I can't wait."

Henry's heart pumped a little faster. "Your mother must be relieved," he said.

"She sure is," Dougie said with a broad smile which immediately changed to a puzzled expression. "Henry, how come you only went to visit Mary before she woke up?"

Henry beat his arms and stamped his feet to keep warm. "Boy, it's enough to skin you out," he said, stalling for time. "The hospital is pretty strict about the number of visitors in the room at one time. Your mother wanted to spend as much time with Mary as possible."

Dougie considered the explanation, a finger to his chin. A smile brightened his face once more. "You'll get to see her plenty when she's home."

No I won't, Henry thought.

"You all right?" Dougie said. "You have a funny look on your face all of a sudden."

"Froze to death, that's all. I'd better get inside."

Dougie swiped away clumps of snow from the bag with a gloved hand. "See you later," he said, and whistled "All Around the Circle" as he walked away.

What I wouldn't give to be happy and worry-free like you right now, Henry thought, and closed the door. He went to the kitchen and reported the good news to his parents.

"That's grand," Alice said. "Poor Mary nearly perished in the fire and her father doesn't know a thing about it. Such a tragedy."

"Serves Charlie right," Tom grumbled. "What kind of man runs out on his wife and two small children?"

"You grew up with him, Dad," Henry said. "Did you think he was capable of that?"

"Not at first. But you don't know about a man until he's tested."

Alice stacked plates in the dishpan. "Thank heavens Mary will make a full recovery," she said. "The darling girl is due some good luck."

Henry ripped apart a slice of ham. "Mary never talks about her father. Not even when he first took off."

"Can't say as I blame her," Tom said. "No father has the right to hurt his family the way Charlie did."

FLORA HELPED MARY WITH HER coat, taking care with her broken shoulder. "Does that hurt?" she said.

"Not too bad," Mary said. Her voice sounded weak.

Flora dressed her daughter with hat, scarf, and gloves like she was a small child. "You can't afford to catch a cold."

Mary dragged the scarf down from her mouth. "I'm smothering, Mom."

Flora took the small suitcase, which held Mary's toothbrush and nightgowns, from the bed. "I called a taxi before I came up."

Nurse Dwyer came into the room with a wheelchair. "Into the chair with you, young woman," she said. "Let's not keep the driver waiting."

Mary started for the door. "I can walk."

"Indeed you won't, my girl." The nurse pushed the wheelchair behind Mary. "I'm the boss around here." There was no teasing evident in her voice. "You'll be dead on your feet before you reach the end of the hall. Get your bottom in this right now."

Mary glanced at her mother. Flora shrugged, a slight smirk playing around the corners of her mouth. "I am a little tired," Mary said, and obeyed the order.

No one spoke on the elevator or on the brief walk to the exit.

Nurse Dwyer wheeled Mary outside, even though she hadn't put a coat on over her uniform. "You take care of yourself," she said softly. "We don't want to see you back here as a patient anytime soon."

"I will. Thank you," Mary said as she climbed into the taxi.

The nurse waved as the car drove away. The tail of her white uniform flapped around her thick legs.

Mary rested her cheek against the cold window. "Nothing's the same anymore," she murmured. "Mrs. Gatherall is gone. And all the other lovely residents. Look at what's happened to me." The taxi skidded halfway down the road and spun around.

Flora grabbed Mary. "Please God we'll make it home in one piece," she said, shielding her daughter with her body. A small car swerved to the right to avoid a collision and plunged into a snowbank.

The taxi slid to a stop, facing the right direction. "It's all right, ladies," the driver said, flipping off his hat to wipe his forehead. "I got her under control." The small car safely disengaged from the snowbank and drove past the taxi. "That's a daily occurrence this winter," the driver said. "It takes a year off my life every time."

The taxi turned a corner at the top of Springdale Street. The last remains of Hull Home beckoned to Mary. Look at me, it seemed to call out. I'm still standing. She turned to her mother. "Why can't this all be a horrible dream?"

Flora searched for a comforting word. None came.

The car continued to the end of the road, turned right, then left, and stopped in front of the Norris house. Mary fumbled with the handle. "I'll get that, miss," the driver said, reaching back.

"I can do it," Mary said, and pushed the door open. She slipped on hidden ice. "Shit," she muttered. Her injured shoulder whacked the side of the car. She bit down on her lip, drawing blood.

Flora paid the fare and rushed to her daughter.

Dougie flew out of the house. "Mary," he called, running toward her with open arms. "I missed you an awful lot."

"Me, too. It's good to be . . ." She paused to catch her breath ". . . out of the hospital."

"Mind her bad shoulder," Flora said as Dougie went to hug Mary.

He stared at her drawn face. "Why do you look so sad?"

"Mary's worn out from the drive home," Flora said. "This is the first time she's been out of bed in days. Let's get her inside so she can lie down."

Dougie held the door open for them. "I have milk heating on the stove to make cocoa for us," he said.

Mary smiled. Her sunken cheeks hardly moved. "You're a good brother," she said, and made her way to the couch, panting slightly. Flora carried Mary's overnight bag to her room.

"Mom said you'll breathe funny until your lungs are completely healed. Right?"

Mary nodded. "I'll be up and about in no time." She held the arm of the couch with a hand to help herself sit down.

"Want me to go tell Henry you're home?" Dougie asked.

Mary smothered a scream. She looked at Dougie's face, alive, happy. Her anger dissolved. "Maybe later," she said. "After I've rested."

Dougie fluffed two pillows behind her back and spread a quilt over her legs. Flora brought in a tray loaded with three steaming mugs, cheese sandwiches, and raisin tea buns. "Eat up, Dougie," she said. "You don't want to be late for school."

He grabbed a sandwich and a mug. "There's some man coming after dinner to talk about what will become of Newfoundland if Canada takes us over." Dougie stuffed half of the sandwich into his mouth. "Brother Gabriel says Confederation will cause us to lose our unique Irish culture."

"Unique culture," Flora said. "That's what we're afraid of throwing away. It's all anyone talks about since this Confederation debate started."

Mary held her cocoa between her hands. She hadn't touched a drop.

"Drink up while it's still hot," Flora said.

Mary's lips had barely touched the rim when she lowered the mug back to her lap.

Dougie's eyes shone like an animal caught in a snare. "Mary, you didn't even taste any. Are . . . are you still sick?"

"The cocoa's too hot," she said, blowing across the top. She took a sip. "That's much better."

Dougie's grin returned in full force. "Good. I was some scared you'd never come home again."

"Off to school with you, my boy," Flora said. "I don't want to hear tell Brother Gabriel brought out the belt for you being late."

Dougie hopped up from the armchair. "See ya when I get home, Mary." Halfway across the room, he turned back to his sister. "You're really all right?"

"Go," Flora said, and waited until her son was out the door to speak again. "Love, is there anything I can do to make you feel better?"

Mary massaged a spot over her right eye. “I know Dougie senses that I’m not all right, Mom. I really did try to hide it from him.”

“You’re the one I’m worried about at the moment.” Flora took the cocoa from Mary. “You have a headache, don’t you?”

“It’s the worst one yet.” Bile gushed up. Mary kicked off the quilt and tried to stand up. “I’m going to be sick.”

“Stay put,” Flora said, and ran to the kitchen for a bucket.

The bile stung the back of Mary’s throat. She swallowed, the sour taste spilling into her nose. She covered her mouth as another wave rumbled through her stomach. “Hurry, Mom.” She sat on the edge of the couch, hunched over, every inch of her shaking. A succession of sharp jabs seared through her broken shoulder.

“Here you go,” Flora said, placing a bucket at her daughter’s feet and a glass of cold water on the coffee table. She held Mary’s hair out of her eyes while she threw up, cleaning her face with a wet face cloth at each short-lived reprieve.

“My chest feels like it’s on fire,” Mary said when her stomach calmed down. She lay back against the pillows. “I’m some glad Dougie . . .” She hiccupped. “. . . wasn’t here to see that.” The rapid drumming in her chest was slowly returning to a normal rate. “He’s worried enough as it is.”

Flora sat down on the coffee table and gave Mary a reassuring smile. “The headaches will get less and less as your time approaches. I went through the same when I carried you and Dougie.”

Mary drank the water, each drop cooling the flames scorching her throat and stomach. “Mom, I didn’t mean to bring shame on you and Dougie.”

“I don’t want to hear any more silly talk like that. A baby is a precious gift. Yours in particular.”

Mary's eyes watered. "Why mine?"

"The doctor said it was a miracle you didn't lose the child. That should tell you something."

Mary rested her bruised shoulder against the side of the couch. "I still don't want Henry to know."

Flora folded her hands on her lap.

"Please, Mom. I've made up my mind."

"Have you really given any consideration to how Henry feels? He doesn't know about the baby. Has he walked away despite every effort on your part to encourage him?" Flora paused briefly. "There's a little tidbit you should know. He went to the hospital numerous times to sit with you, praying you would wake up and be all right." Flora caressed Mary's cheek. "He loves you, my sweet girl. That's why you should tell him he's going to be a father."

Mary moaned. "How can you of all people say that?"

Flora smiled. "I'll always do right by you, Mary."

A FLOOD OF COLD AIR chilled the room. Mary woke, sat up, and looked at the clock over the mantel. She had slept for twenty minutes.

"I'm going to be a father." The voice echoed like a hollow whisper from the depths of a deep well. It was Henry. Dougie stood behind him.

"Oh, no!" Mary cried.

Flora hurried from the kitchen. "Dougie," she snapped, "why aren't you in school?"

"I'm not on the pip, Mom. Honest. The Confederation man had to cancel. Brother Gabriel let us go early." He looked at Mary. "I saw Henry and told him you were home."

"You should've kept your big trap shut," she said, sharply.

Dougie's mouth dropped open.

Flora went to Dougie and led him by the arm. "Your sister is out of sorts today. Don't pay her any heed. Henry and your sister need to talk without us gawking at them."

Henry watched them go down the hall to the kitchen before walking into the room, each step precise, mechanical. "A father," he said, as if he had no idea what the phrase meant. "How long have you known?"

Mary's headache pounded in her ears. "I saw the doctor just before the fire."

"Why didn't you tell me?"

"Mom shouldn't have told you."

"She did the right thing."

Mary pulled the quilt up around her. "How do you feel about it?"

Henry dropped into the armchair facing the couch. "Shocked," he said quietly, and stared down at the floor.

Mary glared at the top of his head. "Shocked," she said with a slight catch to her voice. "That's all?"

"I spent hours thinking about what you said that night outside your house. You said I used you. It winded me."

"I'm sorry you felt slighted," Mary said, her face a canvas of unreadable emotions. "It's what I believed and still do."

"It must've seemed that way when I applied to medical school. In truth, I just didn't think about our relationship."

"You're free to leave Newfoundland anytime." Mary rested trembling fingers on her stomach concealed by the quilt. "I won't burden you with any of the responsibility for this child."

"Please, Mary. Hear me out."

"Like I told you that night. There's nothing left to discuss."

"The fire put my feelings for you in perspective," Henry

said, as if she hadn't spoken. "I understand now what's important to me."

"Don't you see that it doesn't matter? You planned a life that has no room for me."

You've lost weight, Henry thought. You look like a truck ran over you. He sighed. All that hasn't touched your beauty. "We have to get married," he blurted.

Mary glowered at Henry. "I'll marry one day because I want to, not because I have to."

"That's not what I meant."

"There's nothing on this earth that could ever make me part of a shotgun wedding." Mary's voice pitched higher when she continued. "Look where it got my mother." She turned her head into the couch. "Goodbye, Henry."

"Mary, how can you expect me to forget about our baby?"

"Henry," Flora said, her hand gently on his forearm. "You should go for now." He hadn't noticed her come back into the room. "Mary's exhausted."

Henry turned to Flora, his limbs unsteady, the world tumbling away from reality.

"Take some more time to absorb the news about the baby. It's a lot for anyone to take in." Flora smiled. "I promise after a few days' rest, Mary's thoughts will be clearer, more reasonable, and sensible."

Chapter 15

FEBRUARY 21 DAWNED ANOTHER BITTERLY cold day. The first rays of sunlight filtered through the frost-covered window touching Henry's face, wakening him from a dreamless sleep. The plastic wind barrier ballooned out, in, out. Henry sat up. He shivered, jumped out of bed, and dressed. His stomach groaned like a beagle snared in a trap as he hurried downstairs into the warm kitchen.

Tom was halfway through a bowl of porridge he had sprinkled with cinnamon. Alice pulled a handful of bread dough from the pan on the sink, moulded it into an oblong shape, and placed it in the heated pan on the stove. Hot melted butter sizzled and spat into the air. Henry helped himself to a small serving of porridge while he waited for the toutons to fry. He dumped in four spoons of sugar, topped it off with tin milk, and mixed everything together.

"The judicial inquiry into the Hull Home fire is a mere hour away," the radio announcer said.

Alice wiped her hands on her apron and turned up the volume.

"For the last ten days the topic of every conversation everywhere I've gone, including the barbershops, friends' homes, and businesses has been about the tragedy. Even Confederation has taken a back seat, which I never dreamed would be possible. On the way to work I passed by the courthouse to see what was going on. There's already a lineup to the doors. It looks like any newcomers won't stand a chance to get inside."

Alice switched off the radio. "I wish it was all over with," she said.

"It will be soon enough," Tom said. "I've heard real good things about Sir Edward Emerson. He'll get to the bottom of the fire without dragging the session on forever."

Henry finished the porridge. "Gordon Higgins is representing Mr. Hull."

"Figures," Tom said. "Hull can afford one of the most influential lawyers in the city."

"Harry Carter is the Crown prosecutor," Henry continued.

"That's good news, at least. Higgins won't get over Carter's time, that's for sure."

Alice turned over the toutons. Tom and Henry liked them fried to a dark brown. "All the poor residents who died are buried and gone forever. What good will an inquiry do now?"

"Well, love, maybe it'll help save lives in the future. Perhaps even result in passing laws to make fire escapes mandatory."

Alice placed four toutons onto a plate and sat down.

Henry took two, sliced each one down the centre, and drowned the insides with butter and molasses.

"You'd better get going, Henry," Alice said. "Didn't you say that Mr. Carter wanted to see you before the session began?"

"There's time. He's not sure if my testimony is necessary."

Henry picked up his touton. "I hope he doesn't call me." Molasses dripped onto his fingers.

Tom opened the *Daily News*. "If he does, all anyone can ask is that you tell the truth. Is Mary testifying?"

"Yes," Alice said. "Flora told me she's scheduled for this morning."

"I saw her go for a walk up and down the street yesterday," Tom said. "The child's colour is still poor."

Henry shoved the last morsel of touton into his mouth. He rose, still chewing.

Tom gave him a curious look.

Henry turned quickly to conceal the blush rising up his neck. "I must be off," he said, and hurried out of the kitchen. The cold wind struck him like a punch in the face. He looked toward Mary's house. The desire to talk to her, to see her lovely face, tormented him. He wondered if she had already left for the courthouse. She hadn't shown up when he caught the streetcar. People were jammed together in the aisles, and the driver drove past several stops to shouts and calls from unhappy patrons on the street. Most of the passengers disembarked at the courthouse to join the already massive crowd. Henry stood back and watched people push their way inside. As a potential witness, he was admitted through a side entrance.

Everyone scrambled for the scant few rows of seats, the benches creaking as men and women pressed together to make room for others. The floor under their feet was wet from melted snow. Voices electrified the air, a steady hum that slowly diminished when Emerson called the session to order. He sat high up behind the desk. A distinguished-looking man with an honest face, Henry thought. Two policemen stood watch at the back by either side of the door. Henry looked for Mary and spotted her in the last seat with her mother. He caught her eye. She looked away. Without any delay Crown Prosecutor Carter got down to business and called Fire Chief Baker to the witness box.

"Chief Baker," the prosecutor began, his hands behind his back. "Tell us what you saw upon arrival at Hull Home the day of the fire."

Baker faced the spectators, a stoic expression on his face. "Smoke billowed into the sky. People hovered in the windows of the main building, trapped in their rooms, flames licking at their backs. I ordered two ladders up. We saved some of them." He closed his eyes.

Henry counted the seconds before he opened them. Five.

"Unfortunately, several jumped when the flames came too close. The fire and smoke were so intense, my men couldn't get in through the windows to rescue anyone." The chief coughed.

Henry had heard that most of the firemen suffered from a cough since the fire.

"The Annex faired a little better, so I ordered water to be sprayed on it to help control the fire. As soon as the water touched the building, it froze into icicles."

"What happened next, Chief?"

"Fire Chief Cadigan and two firemen had to break in the door to the Annex. They found most of the residents huddled together just inside the door."

"Where did most of the survivors reside?"

"In the Annex. It was the farthest away from the source of the fire."

Emerson excused Baker and called Fire Superintendent Vivian.

"You and Fire Chief Baker made a lengthy inspection of the

Home after the fire was extinguished," the Crown prosecutor said. "Please relate what you encountered."

Superintendent Vivian gripped the box rail and glanced in the direction of Isaac before he began. "It was the most gruesome sight of my entire career," he said. "In the main building, some residents had died in their beds, victims of smoke inhalation." The superintendent's voice kept its professional tone. "Some had rallied enough strength to get one leg to the floor." His face grew more ashen as he recounted the details. "Others were found in a kneeling position, their hands joined in prayer."

The spectators listened. Not a squeak or whisper could be heard.

"The second and third floors were gutted. Water was everywhere. Charred wood and debris of every sort flowed down the stairs. The walls to the majority of rooms had burned down. Icicles hung everywhere, water dripping from them like a rain shower." The superintendent gently touched an earlobe that had been frostbitten during the fire. "Burned furniture, clothing scorched almost to dust lay scattered everywhere. The roof sagged in several places. Most floors were all but destroyed. The kitchen stove was nothing more than a clump of black material." He cast another look at Isaac. "A mattress caught fire when one of my men attempted to remove a deceased resident from it."

"Tragic indeed," Carter said. "You and Mr. Cahill, a city building inspector, inspected Hull Home for safety issues before the fire."

"Yes."

"What were your findings?"

"The condition of the kitchen stove and the lack of fire escapes were my main concerns. I noted that several of the rooms were overcrowded."

Henry glanced back at Mary. Her eyes were fixed on Inspector Vivian, her face grim.

"To your knowledge, Inspector," Carter said, "had the Hulls complied with any of your recommendations?"

"No. The report was published in both local papers. I assumed City Hall would send the Hulls a copy and enforce the required safety regulations. The Department of Health and Welfare proceeded with their own inspection following my report."

A representative from City Council testified next that they were not aware Mr. Hull's establishment had been converted into a nursing home. The Health Department witness claimed the city was responsible for enforcing safety regulations.

"A scandalous situation," the Crown prosecutor said. "It would appear that no official department felt the need to make sure our elderly were looked after properly."

Emerson leaned forward. "To which I wholeheartedly concur," he said.

The spectators applauded.

Gordon Freeman, the stove mechanic, took the witness box and spoke about leaking oil, the number of times he had repaired the stove, and the many occasions he had warned Mr. Hull against tampering with the carburetor.

Henry saw Mary nod in agreement.

Ronald Cave, the man who painted the Home prior to the fire, came next. Carter asked him about the scorch marks behind the stove.

"Well, sir," Cave said, looking at the prosecutor while picking white paint from under his fingernails. "To my recollection, there weren't any scorch marks behind the stove when I painted the kitchen."

Frank Wylie, the businessman who occupied the first floor of the Home, gave his testimony next. He adjusted the lapels of his jacket before answering. "I was sitting at my desk, working away, when I smelled oil. Couldn't believe my eyes when it dripped from the ceiling onto my goods. We had to move a load of boxes and put a bucket under the leak."

Two former residents of Hull Home gave testimony. One said the living conditions were very comfortable, the food healthy and abundant. The other swore the rooms were overcrowded, the food sparse and poorly cooked.

Nurse Jean Baker, dressed to perfection in her uniform with cape and hat, proclaimed the care at the Home second to none. The remaining two nurses agreed the Home was beyond reproach.

At twelve sharp, Emerson called a recess for dinner. Many of the spectators chose to remain so as not to lose their place. Henry headed toward the door. Mrs. Norris smiled at him and followed her daughter outside. Henry saw them descend the many steps at the side of the courthouse which led to Water Street. He turned in the opposite direction and went home.

"How's it going?" Tom asked when the family was seated at the table.

"It's hard to tell. Half the witnesses praise the Home. Half condemn it." Henry paused in his eating. "My impression is that City Hall and the Health Department will share in the blame for the fire with Mr. Hull." He explained what had come out at the inquiry thus far.

"My mother and all the others died horrible deaths because of a group of men in high positions," Alice said. "Men who didn't give a damn about old and sick people."

*

HENRY RETURNED to the courtroom at 1:30 p.m. Mary and her mother had already retaken their seats. The first witness called was Isaac Hull. He wore a brown suit with a brown shirt. His hands were bandaged, injured during the fire. Henry noticed he seemed unsteady as he walked to the witness box.

"Mr. Hull," Carter began. "Do you deny that you tried on numerous occasions to repair the kitchen stove yourself?"

Isaac cleared his throat. "I did a little tinkering, nothing serious."

"What did you do when you discovered the fire in the kitchen?"

"Flames shot up around the kettle and from the back of the stove. The heat was unbearable and the smoke stung my eyes. I couldn't see a thing." Isaac glanced around the room from under heavy brows. "Even so, I tried to get a bucket and fill it with water."

"Did you succeed?"

"No. The fire had spread all through the kitchen." Isaac lowered his head.

"Go on, Mr. Hull."

"I ran to the foot of the stairs and shouted 'fire.' I met Howard Pike and told him to call the Fire Department."

"What did you do then?"

"I . . . I went outside."

A low murmur rippled through the spectators.

Mr. Carter waited for Emerson to bring order to the room. "Tell me, Mr. Hull, why didn't you go upstairs to warn the residents, to help organize a rescue effort?"

Isaac flicked his eyes right and left as if he didn't know where to look. "I was afraid for my life. Although I helped rescue residents from the Annex."

"Is that a fact, Mr. Hull? Fire Chief Baker testified that Fire Chief Cadigan had to break in the door of the Annex in order to remove the residents."

Isaac remained silent.

The Crown prosecutor walked back and forth in front of the witness box. "Why did you not implement the recommendations of the fire inspector?"

Isaac moved around on the chair. "I never received any formal notification from City Hall or the Health Department to do so."

"Did you take it upon yourself to inquire if you should implement fire escapes?"

Isaac seemed to shrink in the chair. "No."

"I have three more witnesses to call," Carter said when Isaac returned to his seat. "The first is Miss Mary Norris, the charwoman at Hull Home."

Henry watched her walk to the witness box, pale, her bad shoulder strapped to her side. Her eyes fell on him, lingering a few seconds. His face burned.

"Miss Norris," the Crown prosecutor said, "you sustained serious injuries in your attempt to rescue residents during the fire, with no thought to your own welfare." He turned to face the spectators, then looked back at Mary. "Very commendable indeed. As you are not yet fully healed, I will endeavour to keep my questions brief and to the point."

Mary produced a weak smile.

"What can you tell me about the condition of the stove at Hull Home?"

Her gaze shot to Mr. Hull. Henry was certain he saw an apology in her expression. Isaac twisted a pencil around and around in his hand.

"It leaked often," Mary said. "Mr. Hull would try to fix it himself. When that didn't work, he called in a mechanic."

"Miss Norris, did you ever 'tinker' with the stove?"

"No. Mr. Hull wouldn't let me."

"Did Mr. Hull do anything else concerning the stove that bothered you?"

"He hung wet dishcloths on the pipe behind the stove to dry them." Mary swayed slightly and grabbed the box rail.

Henry sprang to his feet and was about to run to her when Flora rushed forward.

Emerson turned to the court clerk. "Bring the young lady a glass of water."

The man left and came back almost immediately. Mary drank slowly, swallowing after each sip, and her colour returned.

"Thank you, my dear," Emerson said. "You may step down."

Flora helped her daughter back to her seat.

Henry's heart lurched when his name was called. Carter smiled at him. "You worked as an accountant at Hull Home. Did you ever witness problems with the kitchen stove in the main building?"

"Sometimes you could smell the oil when it leaked. Mr. Freeman was called many times to repair the stove."

"Can you comment on the quality of food served?"

"I only ever ate tea and toast there."

"Your grandmother, Mrs. Dorothy Gatherall, was a resident." Carter paused. "My sympathies on her passing in the fire."

"Thank you," Henry said.

"Did she ever comment on the conditions?"

"Gran, my grandmother, was leaving the Home to come

live with us. She was tired of the same food all the time and wanted a room to herself."

"One final question. In your opinion, was Hull House a good place to reside?"

Henry looked straight at Mary. "There were some good people there."

She blushed and looked down.

Dr. Kennedy took the stand. Henry hadn't noticed him before.

"From what I observed on my weekly visits to the Home," the doctor began, his voice strong and clear, "the tuberculosis patients were well looked after. In my considered opinion, the nurses treated them with care and respect."

"Doctor," Carter said, "do you feel that three nurses were adequate for the number of tubercular and other sick patients in the Home?"

"They worked long, hard hours."

"Would you go so far as to say they were overworked?"

"Yes."

"Thank you. No more questions."

Dr. Kennedy returned to his seat.

Emerson ran his eyes around the room. "A catastrophe certainly brings things out into the open," he said.

Henry looked to Mary once more.

"Before I conclude this inquiry," Emerson went on, "I have a personal statement to make." He directed his gaze to where senior officials from City Hall and the Health Department sat. "I cannot believe that, having the power and the obligation to enforce safety measures, the city chose to do nothing. As for the Department of Health and Welfare, health and welfare should be a practised priority, not simply a title." He gathered up his notes. “I will review the evidence presented with extreme care and consideration, then render my conclusions as to the cause of the fire and those responsible for the needless, tragic loss of so many lives. Good day.”

Chapter 16

TOM ENJOYED A THIRD CUP of tea and a raisin bun. "I wonder how long it'll be before Emerson releases his findings?"

"I don't expect there'll be any surprises," Alice said, hanging up the dishtowel. "There's more than Mr. Hull to blame." She rooted around in the pantry. "I was sure I bought more than one," she muttered.

"What are you looking for?" Tom asked.

"Flour. I wanted to make an apple pie for dinner." Alice closed the long, narrow door and searched all the bottom cupboards. "I could have sworn I bought an extra bag last week when Mr. Royal had the two-for-one sale."

"You must've used it, love. Henry should be back soon. He'll go to the grocery for you."

"I'll go. Do you need any cigarettes?"

"No thanks. I have a half-carton left."

Halfway down the hall, Alice called to her husband. "By the way. Don't budge from that chair while I'm gone," she said. "See you in a few minutes."

"I'm not a youngster," he grumbled back.

"You are while you're on the mend," Alice said sweetly.

Tom picked up the *Daily News* from the table. "More garbage about Confederation," he said, and threw down the paper. He reached into his pocket for a cigarette. The package empty, he stared at the top cupboard next to the pantry where he kept his supply. Tired of having to depend on either his wife or son to even go to the toilet, he reached for his crutches and stood up. He hesitated. Alice would be upset if he attempted anything she considered an unnecessary strain or risk. "Rubbish. I'm a grown man."

He crossed the kitchen on his toes, his fingers almost crushing the handgrips on the crutches. He steadied himself against the pantry and raised a hand to open the cupboard door. As he did, the crutch fell away. Tom lost his balance and tried to grab hold of the door. His missed and knocked a biscuit tin to the floor. The lid popped off and the contents scattered around his feet. "Damn it," he spit out. "I can't even manage a cupboard door." He looked at the wall clock. The grocery store was only around the corner. Alice would be home any minute.

Tom went down on his knees, gathered up the envelopes, and stuffed them in the tin. About to return the can back to the cupboard, the lid popped again. He noticed a return address on an envelope. His pulse hammered while he checked several more, the dates going back ten years.

Tom struggled to keep the crutches from slipping out from under him on his way to the living room. "How could she?" he murmured over and over. He sat and stared out the window. The icicles had thickened to twice their original size. He saw Alice walk up the street with a seven-pound bag of flour under her arm. She stopped to talk with Flora Norris. She smiled a smile which reached her eyes, almost obliterating the traces of grief. His gaze remained on the window even after she had entered.

"Tom," she called. "I saw Bill in the grocery store. There's been another accident with the crane at the dock." She kicked off her boots and went into the living room. "Thank God no one was hurt this time."

Tom kept his head turned toward the window.

"Did you hear me?"

No response.

"Tom, are you all right?"

He pulled out the letters from under the cushion. "What do you think?"

Alice paled, whiter than she had been since the day Dot died. "I . . . I'm sorry," she said.

"Sorry. Is that all you have to say?"

Alice took a deep breath and walked right up to her husband. "You're well aware I've wanted you to hear your brother's side of the story," she said. "I took it upon myself for Henry's sake to get to know Mike in whatever way possible."

"How could you go behind my back like that?"

"I only wanted to reach out to the brother you're afraid to admit you still love."

"I bet he made up all kinds of excuses about why he stayed away."

"No. That was the one subject he wouldn't talk about."

"Mike could always twist words to his advantage."

"For goodness' sake," Alice said. "Read the letters. Your brother isn't the devil you make him out to be." She turned and left before he could answer.

Tom tossed the letters on the coffee table and stared at the pile. He reached for the top envelope, hesitated, then pulled his hand back.

MIKE TOOK OFF THE NAPKIN tucked into his shirt collar and laid it on the empty plate he had been tempted to lick clean as Dr. Kennedy came into the dining room.

"You're late this morning," Mike said.

"My first patient isn't until ten. It's the only day I can catch up on some sleep."

Mike patted his stomach. "Mrs. Simms makes a delicious breakfast."

The doctor smiled. "Don't mention that in her presence. She might ask for a raise."

Mrs. Simms carried in a hefty serving of pancakes. "A raise is a dandy idea," she said, and placed the dish on the table in front of her employer. Her eyes twinkled at Mike. "There's plenty more if you're still hungry, Dr. Gibbs."

"If I touch another bite, I'll have to let out my trousers."

Mrs. Simms graced him with a huge smile. "Give a shout if you change your mind. I'm handy with a needle and thread as well."

The doctor dribbled molasses over two large pancakes. "Seems like you've made a conquest in my housekeeper," he said. "Mind you, she's not easily won over."

Mike held up the morning paper for his friend to see the headline about the inquiry. "How did it go?"

Dr. Kennedy's fork paused midway to his mouth. "It was a terrible business. An awful heartache for the families dredging up what happened, trying to find the cause and assign blame."

"I imagine Henry was called to testify."

"And his girl, Mary Morris. The residents loved her." The

doctor put the knife and fork on his plate as if he had lost his appetite. “She’s not quite physically recovered from the ordeal. Her mental state might be another issue altogether.” He stared at Mike. “She found Alice’s mother seconds after she died of smoke inhalation.”

“The poor girl,” Mike said. “That memory will most likely haunt her for the rest of her days.”

“I’m glad Henry was spared that at least,” Dr. Kennedy said. He dug into the food once more. “Mike, not to change the subject, but you’ve been here for ten days.”

Mike laughed. “Outstayed my welcome, have I?”

“Never, old friend.” The doctor chewed a chunk of pancake, swallowed, and cut off another piece.

Mike supported his chin on the heel of a hand. “I’m waiting for the point you’re taking too much time to make.”

“Time for reasoning with Tom is over. Show him what a headstrong dope he’s been these forty years.” Dr. Kennedy removed the cozy from the teapot and filled his cup. “I know it’ll be somewhat of a shock for him.” He added enough milk to render the tea lukewarm. “Tom’s a grown man. He’ll just have to take everything in stride.”

“I’d rather try to get him to listen to me one more time.” Mike pushed back his chair and stood up. “If that doesn’t work, I’ll take your advice into consideration.”

“Mike, if you want to see your own family anytime soon, I suggest you do more than consider my advice.”

“My wife has given me her blessing to stay as long as it takes.” He took out her picture from an inside pocket. “She’s a lot like Alice. Anyway, I’m going to Tom’s this morning. I’ll fill you in on what happens.”

“Good luck,” Dr. Kennedy said. “You’ll need it,” he

mumbled under his breath when Mike vanished out the door.

"Need what?" Mrs. Simms said.

"Nothing. I was thinking out loud."

MIKE WALKED OUT OF CABOT tower and got into the back of the ABC taxi. His ears were numb, his lips dry. "This has to be the coldest place on earth," he said.

The driver tossed the last of a Camel cigarette out the window, rolled it up, and turned on the ignition. "Where to now?" he asked, glancing in the rear-view mirror. A mixture of smoke and mist from his breath hovered around him. He wound stiff fingers around the steering wheel. "Doesn't take long for the heat to seep out once the car's turned off."

Cabot Tower had been the second stop on the spur-of-the-moment city tour. A ride through The Gut and past Quidi Vidi Lake had been the first. Mike wiped steam from the glass and looked out at the Atlantic Ocean, mere yards beyond the concrete railing used as a protection against the hill's rocky landscape. The sky was a brilliant blue. The sun reflected off the smooth water, undisturbed by wind or waves. He had seen icebergs poke up from the depths like white melted candles the last time he had visited Signal Hill. Several small fishing boats studded the vast expanse.

The taxi rounded the sharp curb at the entrance to the parking lot and started the long, winding ride down Signal Hill. "Buddy, made up your mind yet where you want to go next?"

"Yes, I have. You'll be happy to know it's a house," Mike said, and gave Tom's address.

"It don't bother me none if I have to drive all over the city.

It's freezing to death while you're traipsing around our historic sites is the hard part."

"Can't say as I blame you," Mike said.

"Not to be butting into your business, but you sound like a St. John's man born and bred. Surely you've seen everything by now."

"This is my first time back in forty years."

The car inched down the steep incline, slipping at every sharp curve toward the ditch. "The hill is icy enough to skate on," the driver said. He gazed at Mike in the rear-view mirror. "Not to worry. I've been driving for nigh on fifteen years and never had an accident yet."

"Winter driving on St. John's hills can be treacherous and nerve-racking," Mike said as they neared the bottom. "I'd almost forgotten."

"That's a fact. The horses have an even tougher time of it with their metal shoes and all." The driver passed the Hotel Newfoundland and turned left onto Military Road. Shortly they were abreast of the CLB Armoury on their right. "I'll wager that Joey Smallwood and his crew are in there right now planning the ruination of this country."

"He is determined," Mike said. "I hear a referendum is a few months away."

The driver scowled. "A proper waste of time that'll cost a pretty penny no one can afford in these hard times."

Mike spied a beautiful black horse trotting toward them. "Is that a funeral horse?"

"That it is," the driver said. He stopped, took off his hat, and waited for the funeral procession to pass by.

"It's been years since I've witnessed such a sign of respect for a deceased person."

The taxi man plopped his hat back on and headed toward LeMarchant Road. "I've seen enough funeral processions this week and a half to last me five lifetimes."

The car had warmed up again by the time they arrived at Tom's house. Mike paid the fare along with a sizable tip. "Thanks for your patience," he said, and stayed on the sidewalk, hands in his pockets, until the taxi drove out of sight. He turned to the sound of a door opening.

Alice came out, dressed in her coat and boots. She wore no hat or gloves. "I wondered when you'd be back," she said.

"Tom needed a few days to cool down," Mike said. "Is this a bad time?"

"The mood he's in, there'll never be a good time."

"Has something happened?"

"Nothing I can't handle." Alice looked toward Mary's house. "I was going to drop in on a neighbour. I can do that later and come in with you."

"Would you mind if I spoke to Tom alone?"

"The door's unlocked. Go on in."

Mike turned the handle, hesitated a second, then went inside. The warm air hugged him like a playful child. He sat down on the hall chair to remove his boots.

Tom knelt in front of the fireplace stoking the flames to a roaring fire. "Is that you, Henry?" he said, reaching for a log from the heap in the steel container. Tom crawled back to the armchair and the tea he had left to cool on the side table.

Mike walked into the room without making a sound. "Hello, Tom. How are you?"

Tom's hand shook when he laid the delicate china mug down. Tea slopped over the side. "What the hell are you doing here?" he demanded.

Mike sat down on the couch. “I told you I wouldn't give up.”

Tom soaked up the tea with his white handkerchief. “I don't want to talk to you.”

“Tell me, little brother. Why are you afraid to hear me out? What harm could it do if it turns out you're right about me?”

Tom turned to him. “You're still a master at spinning a situation to your benefit. You haven't changed.”

“Exactly.”

“So you admit it.” Tom glared at Mike. “Now get out and leave me and my family alone.”

“You misunderstand. I haven't changed in any way. I still like to read mystery books, listen to ghost stories on the radio, skate on frozen ponds, be near those I love. “

Tom laughed. “Be near those you love. You're quite the joker, aren't you?”

Mike crossed his legs at the ankles. “From what I've seen, you're the one who's changed. And not for the better.”

“Ah. I see the plan now. Turn the tables on me. Make it appear as if you're the mistreated soul while I'm the louse who doesn't give a damn.” Tom sat up straight. His feet slipped off the stool with a clunk that sent spasms of pain up his calves. “You broke our mother's heart twice.” He fell back into the chair as if worn out. “She was devastated by our father's death and again when you stayed away.”

“I realize how hurt you are.”

“Don't talk to me about hurt.”

“Tom, forty years is a long time to hold tight to a grudge I don't deserve. You've treated me like I don't exist. Well, I do.” Mike uncrossed his legs. “And I'm here to tell you that I've had enough.”

"No one's forcing you to stay. My life has been fine without you."

"I wrote letter after letter to you explaining why I didn't come home for the funerals. I wanted you to come live with me in Toronto after Mom died."

Tom snatched Alice's secret letters from the coffee table and threw them at Mike. "You persuaded Alice to go behind my back."

Mike stared at the letters splayed across the floor. "You haven't confronted her yet?"

"Yes I did."

"And?"

"And nothing. Alice has a mind of her own. She defended her reason for going against my wishes."

The hint of a smile crept across Mike's face. "So you can be reasonable when you want to be. Tom, I love you. My professional life and family life have been blessed, yet there's an emptiness that only you can fill."

Tom looked deep into his brother's eyes. "I can never forgive you for staying away from our parents' funerals." He turned his head away. "Believe it or not, I have tried."

"Is there nothing I can say to change your mind?"

"Nothing." Tom kept his head turned away.

Flames sputtered in the grate when Alice entered the house. "It's enough to blow you away," she called. Her voice was barely heard over the noise of wind as she held fast to the door to keep it from slamming shut. "Tom," she said quietly, "I'm home."

"I'm still here," Mike said.

"Yes," Tom added, "you're in time to see him leave for good."

Alice took off her coat, hung it up, and placed her boots on the rubber mat. She smoothed down her tousled hair and joined the two men. "Dear God," she cried out, hands to her mouth. Her face grey, she stared at Mike.

"Tom," Mike said, "this is the reason I couldn't get home." He stood on one leg. The right leg was amputated just below the knee. A prosthesis lay against the couch. "I didn't want to shock either of you like this."

Tom half rose out of his chair, then dropped back. He looked from his brother to Alice, then back to his brother. Mike sat down and reattached the prosthesis. Not a sound was heard. Even the fire seemed to quiet down in respect for the scene unfolding before it. Alice moved to her husband's side. Tom gaped up at her. She smiled.

Tom finally found his voice. "W . . . what do you mean that's the reason you didn't come home?"

Mike's hand trembled as he ran it through his hair. "The accident occurred on my way to the train station to come home." He closed his eyes briefly before looking at Tom once more. "The roads were slippery from a storm the night before. The taxicab skid down a hill and rolled onto its side. I was trapped. The driver died on the way to the hospital."

Mike stood up and paced in front of the couch. The slight limp was pronounced. "I was unconscious for two days. It took six hours of surgery to save my leg."

"To save your leg," Alice said. "But . . ."

"An infection set in almost immediately," Mike said without looking at anyone. "Two weeks following the first surgery, I had another operation to amputate the lower leg, by now gangrenous. A full week went by after the accident before I was coherent enough to even think properly." He looked at

Tom. "I wrote as soon as I was able. Mom never answered my letter. I couldn't understand why not."

"I'm sorry," Tom said.

"It wasn't your fault. When Mom died I wasn't well enough to travel and wrote asking you to come live with me in Toronto." Mike sat down. "It killed me thinking that she died believing I didn't care about her or Dad." He took a deep breath. "I wrote over and over. Even sent telegrams. Then I began to think that Mom didn't receive my letter. Or maybe she was so upset with me for leaving she wouldn't read it."

"Mom wasn't angry with you," Tom said, his voice almost a whisper. "She was broken-hearted that you had thrown us aside."

"Then my letter didn't arrive."

Mike looked at his brother intently. The fire crackled behind the grate.

Tom swallowed, sick to his stomach.

"I tore it up," he said.

Mike sighed. "I thought it might be something like that."

Alice gasped. "Tom, why did you do such a horrible thing?"

Tom winced, her words stronger than a physical blow. "Because I was a goddamned idiot," he said, and turned to his brother. "Mom was devastated over Dad's sudden death. When the letter came I was convinced it would contain phony excuses why you weren't here."

Mike listened, his head lowered into his hands.

"Oh, Tom," Alice said softly, "your mother deserved better than that from you."

"Mike," Tom said, "I don't know what to say." He raised his eyes to the ceiling, shaking his head over and over. "If I had given the letter to Mom, we would've gone to Toronto. Instead she died of a broken heart and you went through the worst time of your life alone."

Henry came into the room and looked from his father's face to the top of Mike's head. "Mom," he said. "What's going on?"

THE FIRE HAD DIED. THE wind raged outside and the sun was trapped behind a mass of clouds. Henry and Alice had left the two brothers alone. A strangled silence soaked the air.

"Mike," Tom said quietly. "Can you ever forgive me?"

Mike looked up. "I already did forgive you, years ago."

Tom pulled out a handkerchief and blew his nose.

Mike walked over to him. "I came here to get my little brother back. That hasn't changed."

Chapter 17

HENRY WALKED DOWN THE STREET and went around the corner, past the bakery and the tobacconist. He retraced his steps to the bakery. His mother would appreciate a bag of crinkles, a break from making a homemade dessert. About to pull open the door, he turned and headed home. The Norris house seemed to stand out larger than the others as he tried to gather up courage to speak to Mary. He knocked on the front door, his mouth dry, his heart bouncing around in his chest like a Ping-Pong ball. Snow fell around him. Large flakes covered his shoulders and bare head. He tapped once on the door. If Mary answered, he would be turned away without even a hello. Footsteps sounded behind the door, strong, steady. Henry held his breath and waited.

Flora opened the door. "Henry, I thought you might stop off here."

"How did you know?"

"I saw you parade up and down the street."

"Is Mary home? I must talk to her."

"Come in." Flora moved aside for Henry to enter. "She's in the kitchen having a cup of tea."

The snow in Henry's hair melted into his eyes. He wiped it away with his coat sleeve.

"Mary's coming along quite good," Flora said as Henry untied his bootlaces. "The migraines are all but gone."

Henry looked up. "And the baby?"

"No problems so far."

Henry followed Flora through to the kitchen. Mary sat with her back to the door and was looking out the window. "Hello," he said, surprised his voice didn't quaver.

Mary turned her head. "Mom shouldn't have let you in."

Flora gave Henry an encouraging smile and left.

Mary watched her mother go down the hall. "There's nothing left to say."

Henry sat down. "What about the child?" he said.

Mary glared at him. "Don't get comfortable. You're not staying."

"Your mother did the right thing in telling me about the baby."

Mary laughed. "The right thing. That, my son, is a matter of opinion."

"What do you mean?"

"Come on. Henry, look at you. The 'right thing' has you squirming like a trapped rat."

Henry picked at a piece of the torn plastic tablecloth. "Don't you care anymore about what's right and decent?"

Mary stared into her cup. Tea leaves formed a maple-leaf pattern. "Right and decent," she repeated without looking up. "That's simply another way of saying you're willing to do your duty, take responsibility for a mistake."

"I want to be a part of our child's life. I deserve that. He or she deserves that."

Mary didn't reply.

Henry pressed on. "I want to marry you, be a family."

"All you can think about is what is right, what you want," Mary said, her hands clenched like claws. "What about what I want, what I need? I told you I will never be an obligation to you or anyone else."

"Our marriage wouldn't be an obligation. I love you, Mary. I know now that I always have."

Mary flinched. "Lies won't change my mind."

"What can I say or do to convince you I'm telling the truth?"

She lowered her eyes to the cup again. "Nothing. It's too late."

"I won't give up. I can't. You and the baby are too important to me."

Mary peered at him. "Don't you dare tell anyone else. This is my business. I'll deal with it."

Henry glanced over his shoulder as he walked out of the kitchen. Mary had turned back to the window.

Flora saw him to the door. "Give Mary a little more time."

"More time. She rejects me every chance she gets, and it hurts more every time."

"She'll come to realize that you're nothing like her father."

"What if she doesn't?"

"Then we'll have to find another way to break her resolve."

ALICE WALKED TO HENRY'S BEDROOM and stood in the doorway. He had come home an hour ago and gone upstairs without so much as a hello. "There you are. I wasn't sure you were home," she lied.

Henry sat in a chair, his eyes fixed on nothing in

particular. The book he had been reading lay on the floor, cast aside. He gave no indication he was aware of his mother's presence.

"What are you doing up here in the middle of the day?" she said. "Your father's been asking for you."

"I wanted to be alone to think," he said, his voice barely audible.

"About medical school?"

"No."

"About Mary?"

Henry looked at his mother, his expression blank. "Why would you think that?"

"I've been so preoccupied with Mom's death and Mike's visit these few weeks, I failed to notice that Mary hasn't been around much."

"Her injuries kept her away."

"That was true in the beginning. She's been well enough to go out shopping with her mother."

"I guess."

"Henry, you haven't mentioned Mary since the fire. Actually, it's been longer than that." When he didn't speak, Alice continued. "She must be upset about your plans for Canada."

"She was."

"You're saying she's not anymore? Is that what's bothering you?"

"Partly."

"I can see that you don't want to talk right now," Alice said softly. "I'll leave you to your thoughts."

"Mom," Henry said when she reached the door. "I'm sorry. I can't tell you."

"I won't pester you for answers. A question for you, however. How has keeping things inside worked for this family so far?" Alice sighed. "Dinner will be ready in an hour. Uncle Mike and Dr. Kennedy are coming over."

"I'll be down in a little while."

TOM PUT THE *TELEGRAM* DOWN when Alice came downstairs. "Well," he said, "did you find out what's on his mind?"

"He didn't want to discuss it. But I was able to drag out of him that Mary's involved."

"How?" Tom said. "Were they all that serious about each other?" He traced a finger back and forth along one side of his jawline. "Henry started moping around a week ago."

"It has to be something awful," Alice said. "I've never seen him brood like this before."

"Dot would have gotten him to open up," Tom said.

"I know." Alice felt for the locket tucked under her sweater. "She had that way about her, especially with our son. Maybe he'll be in a better mood when Mike gets here."

"Yes," Tom said. "He'll have a ton of questions about Canada."

"It's a good thing Henry will have your brother to look out after him," Alice said. "He'll be lonely enough as it is. Tom, are you really all right with Henry going away to be a doctor?"

"I know what I thought before. But it's all right now. It's more than all right."

"It's good that our son wants to be like Mike and Dr. Kennedy," Alice said. "Two excellent doctors."

"Yes," Tom said. "Dr. Kennedy told me the other night that Mike is considered one of the top orthopaedic surgeons in

Canada. He's even been offered loads of money to work in the United States but refuses to go."

Alice flashed her own smile of approval. "Very impressive," she said.

"He's still down-to-earth. Our Henry will follow in his footsteps."

Alice hummed softly, flattening pastry with a rolling pin until it was paper-thin, the way Tom and Mike both liked. Having cut up apples and sugar and added a teaspoon of cinnamon, she put the finished product in the oven. The aroma of apple pie cooking sailed through the house by the time the two supper guests arrived.

Already on his way down the stairs, Henry answered the door on the first knock.

"My boy," Dr. Kennedy said, "a drink of screech will knock the chill right out of my arthritic bones."

Mike blew on his hands to restart circulation. "Good idea."

Henry poured the drinks and sat with the men while they chatted about the Confederation campaign.

Tom drank half the glass in one shot. "No offence, Mike, but Newfoundland is better off staying a separate country with our own laws. There's no telling what sort of strange rules Canada might impose."

"There would be many changes," Mike agreed. "Whether bad or good would depend on if you're open to change."

Alice called them to supper. "Mike," she said when they were all seated, "Tom told me you used to love fish and brewis with scruncheons."

Mike sucked on a squared piece of fried pork fat. "There is no food on earth than can compare with it," he said. "My wife cringes every time I fry up a batch. She won't give it a try."

Dr. Kennedy drizzled fat over his brewis. "Good old Newfoundland food was the one thing I missed the most when I was away to study medicine."

"And Irish Newfoundland music," Mike said. "Always makes you want to get up and do a jig."

Dr. Kennedy smiled, reflecting on long-ago memories. "The minute I opened my mouth, everyone assumed I came from Ireland. I allowed the ladies to believe that." He grinned. "For a while, anyway."

"Might as well have been Ireland," Mike said. "No one had ever heard of Newfoundland, let alone knew where it was located."

Alice added extra fried onions to her fish and brewis. "Fred Russell, the bakery man, visited Toronto once and told me it was a huge place," she said, a worried look in her eyes. "It must've taken some getting used to."

"It did," Mike said. "Once you get busy with school and books, your world revolves around the university." He forked a chunk of brewis into his mouth. "The main differences I noticed were the number of people and the buildings. Ten, fifteen storeys high, all made of concrete. Houses as well were made of brick, none of the bright colours like the wooden homes here."

"Must look awful dull," Alice said.

Tom slopped vinegar all over his supper. "Sounds like a whole other world," he said.

"It grows on you with enough time," Mike said.

"And," Dr. Kennedy added, "the summers are longer and warmer. The winters much colder. Except this winter, of course."

Alice tried not to stare at Henry and draw attention to

him. He sat quietly, eating like it was a practised exercise that required no focus.

"Gathering fairy dust, Alice?" Tom touched her arm. "What are you thinking about?"

She started. "Sorry, love. What did you say?"

Tom chuckled. "You left us for a while there."

Dr. Kennedy exchanged a look with Alice. "I'd say your wife was thinking about Henry's imminent departure. All mothers fret about a child leaving home."

Alice sneaked another glance at her son. She was sure he hadn't heard a word. "You're absolutely right, Doctor," she said. "Then again, you've gone through the mixed emotions of a child leaving home three times."

"Don't worry," Mike said. "I'll take good care of my nephew. He can stay with me as long as he likes."

Alice drank a mouthful of water. "That's very good of you, Mike. Will your wife mind having a young man underfoot?"

"Not in the least. Our two sons are married. Lilah will be in her glory having someone other than me to fuss over."

Tom turned to Henry. "What do you think of that?"

"Uncle Mike, I appreciate your generous offer." He shoved food around his plate. "I can't take you up on it."

"Why not?" Tom said.

Henry took a deep breath. "I've changed my mind about school."

Dr. Kennedy stuck a finger in his ear as if to clear away the wax. "Did I hear you correctly?"

Tom's face flushed a deep red. "What's all this about, Henry?"

Alice looked at her husband with sad eyes. "Please don't be angry with him."

"Love, I'm confused, not angry. Henry, I've been hard on you about school. That's behind us now. Medical school is a grand idea."

Mike wiped his mouth with his napkin. "Why the sudden change of heart?" he said quietly.

Henry looked from one to the other. "I can't say." He pushed back his chair and rushed out of the kitchen. The front door opened and closed.

Tom's mouth hung open. "What in the hell was that about? He was over the moon about medical school and being a doctor."

Alice stared around the table. "I know Mary's been on his mind since the fire."

"It's most likely a case of nerves," Mike said. "Moving to a new country is a daunting step for someone who's never been away from home before."

"I don't think that's it," Tom said. The creases in his forehead deepened. "I know my son. Something really serious has happened. Something so awful he can't tell us."

Dr. Kennedy rubbed his chin. "Henry hasn't said a word to me about any kind of problem."

Alice glanced toward Dot's empty chair. "He would've confided in Mom and she'd have the problem sorted out by now."

"I wish I'd had the chance to meet her," Mike said.

Tom sighed. "A fine woman who took no nonsense," he said. "Henry must miss her."

Alice plastered a smile on her face. "Homemade apple pie for dessert," she said. "Hope you all saved room for it."

"Lovely," Dr. Kennedy said. "I'll have an extra-large slice." He turned to Mike.

"Don't let on to Mrs. Simms. The woman would have my head if I stuff myself with sweets."

Forced laughter around the table soon died.

Alice cut the pie and everyone watched the steam rise from the delicious, steaming dessert.

Chapter 18

MARY YAWNED AND TURNED ONTO her side. She winced as her broken shoulder made contact with the mattress. Pain shot across her collarbone and down her arm. She turned onto her back and looked at the alarm clock. For most of the night, she had been awake thinking about Henry's visit. He was racked with guilt and willing to do anything to appease his conscience. She leaned on her good elbow trying to sit up. Another jab of pain. The room spun, nausea assaulted her without warning. "Not again," she groaned, swinging her legs over the side of the bed. Her stomach gurgled, the contents threatening to gush up to her throat. She swallowed and the sensation passed.

Her feet touched the canvas floor. So cold. Sweat broke out on her neck, her arms, the back of her knees. She bolted upright, whipped open the bedroom door, and ran for the bathroom. The uneven floor creaked like scared mice as she fled down the hall.

Dougie burst out of his room. "Mary, what's the matter?"

She dashed past him.

"Mom," Dougie shouted. "Mary's sick." He flew after his sister.

She dropped to her knees in front of the toilet and vomited. Her tongue stung. Specks of bile spattered on her nightgown and clung to her hair. The sour smell saturated the air. Dougie gagged.

Mary fell back on her heels. "Dougie," she said, dragging a hand over her mouth. "Wet a face cloth for me."

Flora appeared behind her son. "Dougie, get dressed. You'll be late for your paper route."

"Oh, God," Mary wailed, and reached for the toilet. Tears flowed down her cheeks as her stomach emptied.

Flora soaked a cloth in icy cold water and pressed it to her daughter's forehead.

Dougie lingered in the hall. "What's the matter with her?" he said, eyes large.

Mary's head hung over the toilet. Her chest hurt. Her broken shoulder smarted like it had been rammed into a brick wall. She lowered the lid and flushed the toilet.

Flora turned to her son. "I promise your sister will be all right."

Dougie stared at Mary's grey complexion. "But she's throwing up some lot lately."

Flora twirled Dougie around and, with hands on his shoulders, directed him to his bedroom. She opened the heavy, beige curtains. The sky was overcast and very little light came in.

"Mom. Please tell me the truth. Is Mary going to get better, or . . ." With a big toe, he poked at a spot on the floor only he saw. "Is she going to die?"

Flora took his face in her hands. "Throwing up is normal for what ails her. It'll pass and she'll be back to her old self."

Dougie held his mother's gaze, his expression serious, older. "Mom, would you tell me if she wasn't going to be all right?"

"I promise to never keep anything that important from you." Flora tousled his hair. "Now get dressed," she said, closing the door on the way out.

Mary wobbled down the hall. She supported herself with a hand on the wall. The floor rose up. A few more steps to go, she thought, and put a foot forward. Her knees gave way.

"You poor dear," Flora said, catching her daughter. "Let's get you back to your room in one piece."

"Mom," Mary moaned. "Will this sickness ever end?"

"Sadly, you take after me in this instance."

Mary sat on the edge of the bed and nursed her shoulder. "Poor Dougie," she said. "He's some worried about me."

Flora sat next to her daughter. "He is," she said. "Furthermore, it's not fair to him."

"Mom," she sobbed. "I can't take you being mad at me."

"I'm not mad. I'm concerned about you and about the effect this situation is having on you and your brother."

"Mom, I didn't get pregnant on purpose."

"For heaven's sake, love, that's not what I meant. How long do you intend to hide it from Dougie? From everyone?"

"I don't know. I can't seem to sort anything out."

"Love, time is running out. Soon the decision to reveal your big secret will be out of your control." Flora wiped away a few traces of vomit from her daughter's face with the tail of her apron and helped her lie down. "Henry has the right to know where he stands." She sighed and left the room.

When Mary heard her mother go down the stairs, she buried her head under the covers and wept.

Dougie slurped tea from a saucer as he looked across the table at his mother. He laid the tea down and dug into the porridge. "Mom, why does Mary get mad every time I bring up Henry?"

"Mary gets testy very easily since the fire. She's been through a hard time." Flora cut a slice of toast into four pieces. "It's going to take time for her to come 'round."

Dougie ran his spoon through the thick, milky oatmeal, and then let it go against the side of the bowl with a slight clink. "Henry never comes by anymore." He dropped his chin into his hand. "Mary never talks about him, not even when Mrs. Gibbs is here."

"Like I explained before, she—"

"Mom," Dougie said, cutting her off. "I'm almost thirteen, not a youngster anymore. I know you and Mary are keeping something real important from me." He frowned. "It must involve Henry."

Flora opened her mouth to deny the statement.

"I deserve the truth," Dougie said. He closed his eyes and ran a hand through his hair.

Flora stared at the boy who was nearly as tall as a man. "Your father used to do that," she murmured, and took a deep breath. "You're right, Dougie. Mary does have a . . ." she paused to consider the right word. " . . . situation she doesn't want you to know about yet. I can promise you that your sister's health isn't at risk."

"Then why is she throwing up all the time?"

"That will pass."

"Johnnie Smith told me last year his sister used to throw up all the time for a couple of months." Dougie lifted the spoon in and out of the porridge.

"What are you getting at?" Flora said.

"Mom, I might be young, but I'm not stupid." He pushed the bowl of oatmeal away. "I have to go deliver the papers now. I'll finish breakfast later." He stopped at the kitchen door. "You and Mary can trust me." Without giving his mother a chance to respond, he hurried down the hall.

Mary shuffled into the kitchen, poured tea, and joined her mother. Flora watched her add sugar and milk, then stir and taste the hot liquid.

"Mom, you're awfully quiet."

"Dougie is worried to death about you. He's questioned all the excuses we're giving for you being sick."

Mary almost dropped her cup. "Please, Mom. I can't bear for him to know."

"I'll make a batch of pancakes," Flora said, and went to the cupboard. She took down a mixing bowl. "Your little brother isn't so little anymore."

Mary trembled all over. "What does that mean?"

"I think Dougie has figured out that you're pregnant and that Henry is the father."

"Oh, God, Mom. He might tell Henry's parents. We must warn him to keep quiet."

"Love, your brother is becoming a fine young man and more sensible than either of us give him credit for. He's concerned about you." Flora measured out flour and butter. "He's ready to hear the truth."

Mary moved on the chair like she had spent hours sitting on the hard surface. "I'll wait till after school," she said. "It'll give me time to think of the best way to explain everything to him."

"He won't understand why you're pushing Henry away. He's like a big brother to Dougie."

"Don't you think I know that?"

Flora cracked two eggs into the bowl. One contained a blood spot. "Not to worry, love. Dougie will keep your secret if that's truly what you want." She added water and whipped the mixture with a fork. The blood spot blended in with the creamy liquid. "Henry's parents will have to be told."

"Our money will run out soon," Mary said. "I'll look for work as soon as my shoulder is better."

"There's no rush. I have a job."

"What? When did that happen?"

"I start work next week at Bowring's in the dress department."

"Oh, God, Mom. It's all my fault you're forced out to work."

Flora spooned the pancake mixture into the frying pan. "No such thing," she said. "I worked outside the home before I married and rather liked it."

The smell of bacon fat made Mary's stomach churn. She covered her mouth with a hand towel.

"Besides," Flora went on, "I'm looking forward to meeting new people and earning a wage again." She smiled. "There's not enough here to keep me busy all day."

Mary reached for her cup. The tea had gone cold. "You're saying that so I won't feel bad."

Flora flipped over a pancake. "Indeed I'm not. I can't wait."

"Did you tell Dougie?"

"Yesterday morning. He thinks it's a grand idea."

"He never said a word to me."

"Which proves he can keep a secret when asked."

"Mom, I can't believe how relaxed you are about my mess-up."

Flora slid the cooked pancakes onto a plate and dunked the

frying pan into cold water. It hissed. The noise slowly faded. "I learned years ago to take life in stride. Worry never helps." She placed the pancakes in front of Mary. "We coped when your father took off. We'll do it again. Now eat. I don't want you getting sick on me."

Mary cut off a tiny portion of pancake, not bothering to smother it in molasses.

Flora untied her apron and sat down. "What are you going to do about the baby?"

Mary shrugged her shoulders, biting down on her bottom lip.

"Time is getting on, love."

Mary didn't speak.

Flora cleared her throat and forced sternness into her voice. "An unwed mother is not permitted to give birth in any of the hospitals. You'll have to go to the home operated by the Salvation Army. They'll talk to you about giving the baby up for adoption." She paused. "Have you thought about that?"

Mary's hand shook as she raised it to her forehead. "I've done nothing else since I found out."

"I hate to pester you, love, but it's high time to think long and hard about the future."

TOM AND MIKE SAT IN matching armchairs Dot had given the family as a Christmas gift five years earlier. Each man had a drink of screech. The flames in the fireplace, the only source of light in the room, licked at the grate, spitting and hissing like tomcats in a fight.

Tom rested his glass on his knee with one hand. "I don't know what to make of Henry lately. Becoming a doctor was all he could talk about since he was a small boy."

Mike swallowed a mouthful of his drink. "I spoke to him this morning. All he would say was that something more important has come his way."

"If it's so damned important, why's he acting like the world's about to crumble into ashes?" Tom scratched his nose. "He hasn't been the same since the fire."

"Henry has a few more months before school starts. If he changes his mind, call and let me know."

Tom stared at his glass, swishing the contents around and around. A little splashed out onto his hand. He didn't appear to notice. "Life was so much simpler when Henry was a youngster." A flicker of sadness glazed over his eyes. "And when Dot was here."

Mike smiled. "Frankie told me she stood for no nonsense."

Tom simply sighed.

"I heard an interesting thing," Mike said to cut through the sombre mood. "The date for the referendum vote on Confederation is set for the third of June. The campaign will really pick up speed now."

Tom's head shot up. "What rot! We're doing fine on our own."

"I'm not sure about that," Mike said.

"You're out of touch with Newfoundland. You've been in a different country."

"Not for long!"

"Don't start that again."

Mike grinned. "By the time the vote rolls around, you'll be one of Smallwood's strongest supporters."

Tom gulped down the last of his drink. "Dr. Kennedy is late," he said. "I hope he wasn't called out on an emergency. The pease pudding will be dryer than parchment paper if it's kept too long."

Mike stood, stretched his legs, and walked to the fireplace. “Maybe Frankie will find a way to get to the bottom of Henry’s problem.” He leaned against the mantel and looked out the window. “I’ve never seen so many icicles in all my life. You can hardly see the street.”

“Henry started work as an accountant at Newfoundland Margarine today,” Tom said as if he hadn’t heard his brother. “It’s good honest work, but it’s not what Henry wants for the rest of his life. I wish he’d tell us what’s gnawing at him.”

“Speaking of Henry,” Mike said, indicating the window with a nod of his head, “here he comes.”

HENRY WALKED UP THE STREET, hands in his pockets, his head held high. He went to the Norris house and knocked.

“Hello, Henry,” Flora said. “Come in. It’s nice to see you again.”

“Thank you, Mrs. Norris.”

“How was your first day at the butter factory?”

“Good,” Henry said, aware his mother kept her friend up to date.

“Mary’s in her room having a rest.”

“Oh,” Henry said, his voice heavy with disappointment. “I’ll drop back another time.”

“Never you mind that. It’s time she came down for supper.” Flora turned toward the kitchen. “See yourself up.”

Henry mounted the steps two at a time and trod softly down the hall. The floor creaked. He knocked, waited, then entered. Mary lay facing the door, a pillow cushioned under her broken shoulder. A checkered quilt covered her to the waist. Her eyes were closed, a hand tucked under a cheek. Henry noticed the dark circles, emphasizing her paleness. “Mary,” he whispered.

She mumbled something he couldn't make out. Her lids fluttered open. "Henry. Why won't you leave me be?"

A knot twisted tighter in his stomach. "All I ask is that you hear me out. Really listen to what I have to say."

Mary sat up. The moon's glow cast her face in shadows. "If I do, will you leave?"

Henry remained where he was. "Yes."

"All right. Though it'll be a waste of time. You've already said everything there is to say."

"I've decided to forget about medical school."

Mary fell back against the headboard. "I didn't ask you to do that, so don't put the responsibility for that on me."

"It's my choice, Mary. One that I make without regrets." Henry took a step into the room. "The fire put my life in perspective."

"Henry, please. That's enough."

"Let me finish. You and the baby are more important to me than being a doctor." Henry moved forward another step. "Before the fire, I didn't consider you. I know now what's in my heart." He smiled. "I want you and the baby."

Mary looked away. "Please, Henry." She stopped talking when the front door opened. They listened to Dougie stamp his feet on the front mat and call out asking what was for supper. Henry inched closer to the bed. "You can turn me away as many times as you want. I'll keep coming back. We can have a good life together."

Mary's expression was unreadable. "Are you done?"

Henry stood tall. "For the time being."

"You keep saying the fire brought on your big turnaround. If I wasn't pregnant, would you be here wanting me to marry you?"

"Even if you weren't pregnant, I'd be asking you to marry me."

Mary laughed. "Sidestepping the issue is a good ploy. No one can ever accuse you of being dim-witted." She sighed, exhausted. "Henry, for the last time, forget about me."

"No," was all he said before walking out of the room. "Because I love you," he muttered under his breath in the hallway.

Flora poked her head in Mary's bedroom as soon as Henry had gone. "He has a point," she said. "If you weren't in the family way you would marry him."

Mary stared at her mother. "How can you say that?"

"Don't bother to deny it," Flora said with a wave of her hand. "Your face says it all."

Chapter 19

ALICE SAT AT THE KITCHEN table, turning the pages of the family photo album.

Tom stood in the door leaning heavily on his crutches. "Are you ready, love?" he said softly. "Mike's waiting out front with Henry."

Alice ran a finger across the picture of her mother snapped on Christmas morning. Dot was smiling, unaware that Tom had taken her picture. She held the pearl necklace Alice had scrimped and saved a whole year to buy. Alice kissed the photo, closed the book, and stood up like it was a monumental effort. "I'm as ready as I'll ever be."

Tom moved toward his wife. "Henry picked up the flowers for Dot's grave."

"Good," Alice said. "Carnations were her favourite. Remember how she liked to have them in her room at the Home?" A shadow passed over her face. "That's the only birthday present I can give her now." She clasped the locket to her heart and returned it to the inside of her sweater.

Alice walked behind Tom down the hall. She hesitated

when he opened the door. “I don’t know if I can bear to see the grave.” She leaned against the wall. “It’s terrible that I haven’t gone since the funeral.”

Tom smiled. “Dot will understand if you’re not ready.” He kissed the top of her head. “Are you all right?”

“I’m being silly,” she said. “Let’s go.” The sun shone and the wind was quiet. The temperature had risen by five degrees.

Tom grinned. “I bet Dot arranged this lovely day just for you, Alice.”

Alice nodded, the hint of a smile on her face.

Mike sat in the driver’s seat of Dr. Kennedy’s Buick and watched his brother and sister-in-law walk toward the car. Tom’s face was drawn. It suddenly occurred to Mike the depth of the love that Tom had felt for his mother-in-law.

Henry helped his father into the front passenger seat. Alice joined her son in the back seat. No one spoke on the drive to the cemetery. Mike turned in to the main gate off the boulevard and parked as close to the gravesite as possible. Tom struggled with his crutches, careful not to slip on the pathway and over the hard-packed snow.

Alice hesitated as they approached Dot’s grave.

“You can do this,” Tom said.

Alice sighed, and moved to the gravesite, and placed the carnations, neatly arranged in a pale blue vase, on the hard snow beside a bouquet of fresh, white carnations. “Those must be from Father Whitten,” she said. “He always gave Mom those for a special occasion.”

Henry picked up a stray white petal and placed it with the others. “I ran into Father Whitten outside the butter factory yesterday. He’d just come from visiting Gran.”

Alice stared at the black marble headstone placed on her

father's grave when she was a child, the space slotted for Dot's name now filled in. "Happy birthday, Mom."

Tom and Mike stayed a little to the side and back a few steps. "I talked to Lilah last night and asked her to come for a visit," Mike said, his voice low. "She arrives the day after tomorrow."

"Alice will like that," Tom said. "It'll give her something to look forward to."

"Lilah's been after me for years to show her where I grew up." Mike looked sideways at Tom. "She's anxious to meet the man who's even more stubborn than me." His gaze drifted down at the lake. "We had some good times at the Regatta, didn't we?"

"We sure . . . what the hell is he doing here?" Tom said, his eyes on a man walking through the lower entrance, his head held high.

"Who is it?" Mike asked.

"Isaac Hull," Tom almost spat out. "As far as I'm concerned, he's the man who killed Dot and all the others."

"He looks so ordinary," Mike said.

Henry turned just as Isaac reached the group. "Hello, Mr. Hull," he said. "I'm surprised to see you here."

"I came to pay my respects to the residents we lost in the fire." Isaac nodded to Alice. "Mrs. Gatherall was certainly one of the finest women in the Home. My wife and I miss her wit and charm."

Tom laughed out loud. "Pay your respects! You don't know the meaning of the word. I doubt any of those killed would want you here."

Isaac stood to his full height. "Those are harsh words, Mr. Gibbs," he said. "And I might add that you do not have the right to speak for people you never knew."

"Maybe if you'd been man enough to stay and organize a rescue, some of the dead would still be alive." Tom's hands tightened on his crutches. "Instead an old woman and a slip of a girl took on that responsibility for you."

Alice hurried to her husband's side. "Tom, please let it go."

"Look here, Mr. Gibbs," Isaac said. "The possibility of a fire never once crossed my mind. That's why there wasn't any firefighting equipment at the Home." He glanced at Henry as if seeking support, then looked back to Tom. "No one saw fit to inform me that some safety conditions could have been improved upon."

Tom looked Isaac up and down, as if he found the sight of him distasteful. "Don't try and sell that bill of goods to me," he said. "If you'd truly cared about those old and sick people you would've made sure they were safe."

"You know absolutely nothing about me and therefore have no idea about what I would or would not have done. I'm late for an appointment." Isaac turned and walked back the way he had come.

"Tom," Alice said. "You were a tad hard on him."

Henry stared after his former employer. "I'm not sure I agree," he said. "Mary warned him over and over about the stove. He ignored her every time."

Mike looked down to the road. Isaac got in a car and drove away. "The man did come across as if he didn't have anything to be ashamed of," he said. "Do you think it's possible Mr. Hull is harder on himself than he's willing to admit?"

"Right," Tom sneered. "And I'll be able to run around the lake tomorrow."

Alice shook her head. "All this arguing is useless," she said. "No matter who's at fault, nothing anyone says or does will bring Mom and the others back. I don't want to spend good energy on resentment or hatred." She drew her arm through her husband's. "Tom, you know that Mom would agree with me."

He looked away, but not before Mike saw a spark of grief dull his eyes.

Henry blessed himself. "We best get a move on," he said, "if we want to be on time for dinner at Dr. Kennedy's house."

"Believe me," Mike said with an exaggerated moan. "Mrs. Simms will give us all a tongue banging if we're even a minute late."

MARY SAT BACK INTO THE rocker, her head resting on the wooden spindles. Light from the moon glowed like an electric bulb in a star-rippled sky. Despite the thick quilt tucked around her legs and shoulders, she was cold. Her breath transformed into a grey mist with every exhalation. The headache that had awakened her at dawn had finally subsided. Hunger gnawed at her stomach, stimulated even more by the smell of baking bread, and for the first time all day she felt well enough to eat. She threw off the quilt and was about to stand up when the sound of a car caught her attention.

Dr. Kennedy chugged to a stop in front of the Gibbs house and turned off the motor. Henry helped his father out of the car while Mrs. Gibbs, the doctor, and a man Mary had never seen before headed toward the front door. She studied the stranger. Tall, broad-shouldered, dark-haired. Alice said something to him and he smiled. His eyes seemed to light up. He must be the deserter brother, she thought.

Mike Gibbs looked up and smiled at Mary. Startled, she turned away from the window.

Dougie stood in the doorway, motionless, his face hidden in shadows. "Mom said Mr. Gibbs was wrong about his brother the same way you're wrong about Henry."

"You'll understand why I feel the way I do in a few years," Mary said in a weary voice.

Dougie shifted to the side and his face became visible. "Sometimes I think I understand better than you do," he said, and left.

Mary looked back out the window. The street was empty, looking lonely without the people to keep it company.

Flora came into the bedroom. Mary's arms were limp at her side, blonde hair hanging down over her face. "Supper's ready," Flora said with a cheery smile. "Stew with dumplings."

Mary rolled her head along the back of the rocker to gaze at her mother. "It smells good," she said, a flat tone to her voice. She stood up. The quilt fell to the floor. "Dougie was just here. He thinks I'm being mean to Henry."

"Unfair is a better word," Flora said.

Mary's hand went to her stomach. "Mom, you more than anyone shouldn't want me to marry Henry under these circumstances."

"Love," Flora said softly, "we've talked about this. You know good and well where I stand. Supper's on the table."

Mary folded the quilt and laid it at the foot of the bed. The hunger had fled, replaced with an empty ache. At the bottom of the stairs, a wave of cramps stabbed at her stomach. Sweat broke out on her brow and she fell to her knees, her arms and legs heavier than barrels filled with oil. "Mom," she tried to cry out. Only a rush of air sounded. Another spasm of pain drove her into a fetal position. "Mom," she tried again, dragging herself down the hall.

Flora passed by the kitchen door. "Sweet Jesus," she cried, and rushed to her daughter.

Dougie jumped up from the table and ran after his mother.

"The pain's some bad," Mary gasped, both hands pressed to her stomach.

"Dr. Kennedy's next door," Dougie said, and bolted outside in his slippers.

The cold air washed over Mary. She shivered.

Flora knelt next to her. "It's all right, love," she said, smoothing sweat-soaked hair away from Mary's forehead.

"The baby," Mary cried. "The baby has to be all right."

Henry came through the door. His eyes mirrored the fear on Mary's face. Dr. Kennedy came next, his coat open, a medical bag in one hand. "Goodness me," he said at the sight of Mary sprawled out like a sack of potatoes on the floor.

"It's my stomach," she whispered through the pain.

"Henry," the doctor said without looking at him. "Get Mary to the chesterfield."

Henry gently lifted her up. She cried out. "I'm sorry," he murmured as he carried her to the living room.

The doctor shed his coat before ordering everyone out.

Flora looked her daughter squarely in the eyes. "He needs to know everything."

Henry didn't budge.

Flora took him by the arm. "Come along. Mary's in good hands."

Dr. Kennedy waited until they were alone to speak. "Dougie said something about you collapsing with severe stomach pains."

"Yes. It's not so bad now."

The doctor took her blood pressure and pulse. "Both a little high, but nothing too serious. Now what was Flora talking about?"

Mary sat up with the doctor's assistance. She blushed and lowered her eyes. "I . . . I'm in the family way."

"I see," the doctor said, as if the revelation was no surprise. He closed the medical bag. "Has there been any spotting?"

Mary shook her head.

"Good. Good."

"Dr. Kennedy, this is the first time anything like this has happened. Will the baby be all right?"

"That, my dear, depends on you."

Mary stared at him. "On me?"

"Worry can kill even the most healthy among us." Dr. Kennedy sat down beside his patient. "To have a healthy baby you must eat right and give up worrying. You're whiter than a bleached sheet and I'd guess you've lost at least eight or nine pounds."

Mary's bottom lip trembled. "It hasn't been easy for me."

"So that's why the boy changed his mind about medical school." The doctor pulled on his ear. "His parents are awfully concerned about him."

"Please," Mary said. "I'm too tired to talk any more."

"Eat something, then go straight to bed. If there's any more cramping, call me right away." He gave a reassuring smile. "It isn't the end of the world, Mary. I can assure you that."

THE NEXT MORNING, HENRY WENT to check on Mary. Dougie bounded up the sidewalk, the empty newspaper bag slung over his shoulder. "Hi, Henry," he said, jiggling coins in his pocket. "I got ten pennies in tips." He hopped up onto the front step. "Come on in. Mary should be up by now."

"How is she? I was some worried about her and the—"

"I know about the baby," Dougie said. "Mary didn't touch a bite again last night. Mom was in and out of her room half the night." His voice took on a lighter tone when he continued. "I was some glad to see her sound asleep when I got up this morning."

"She's having a hard time of it," Henry said.

Flora met them in the hall. "Dougie, your breakfast is ready." She looked at Henry. "Mary's in bed. She had a bad night."

Disappointment registered on Henry's face. "I was hoping to see her."

"Henry, tell me the God's honest truth. Why do you want to marry my daughter?"

"To give our baby a proper name. My name." He looked at Mrs. Norris with a clear, steady gaze. "Most important of all, because I love her more than I believed possible."

"Just as I thought," Flora said. "Just as I thought." She smiled, yet it didn't brighten her face. "Mary's awake. Go on up."

Henry's heart began to gallop faster than a frightened horse as he climbed the stairs. He walked down the hall to her room, rapped on the door, and opened it before Mary could object to him coming in.

She lay back against the pillows, milky white, her cheeks sunken. "Henry, please leave me alone."

"I can't. I won't," he said, moving to the bed.

Mary stared at him, unblinking. "You don't have to worry about the baby any more," she said, her voice a hollow whisper.

"That's easier said than done. What kind of man would I be to walk away from you, from our baby?"

Mary sank into the bed and pulled the covers to her neck. "That obligation is gone."

Henry felt his knees weaken and held onto the bedpost for support. "What do you mean?"

"I miscarried last night. The baby's gone." She turned toward the window. Clouds gathered on the horizon. "You don't have to marry me now."

Henry fell into the rocking chair. "It can't be true." He dropped his head into his hands. "Oh, God. It can't be true."

"I want to be alone," Mary said.

"I love you," Henry said, and ran a hand through his hair. "You'll never know how much I wanted our baby."

Chapter 20

MIKE AND TOM SAT IN front of the fireplace, each smoking a Camel cigarette. Tom puffed out perfectly shaped rings which disintegrated as they floated to the ceiling.

"I've never been able to get the hang of that," Mike said, attempting to blow out a circle. A mushroom cloud formed and flattened almost immediately.

Tom grinned. "It's a natural-born talent," he said. "Either you have it or you don't." His grin faded. "Mike, you haven't truly met the real Henry yet."

"He's on your mind a lot lately."

"Normally he's the kind of person who sees the bright side of things. If he wants something, nothing gets in his way." Tom sighed. "He's seems to have given up."

Alice stood in the entrance to the living room, looking at the grandfather clock. "I don't know what's keeping Henry," she said, turning her eyes to the window. "He should've been here twenty minutes ago."

The front door opened. "Henry," Alice said. "Where were you? I was beginning to worry."

He stared in his mother's direction, yet seemed to look through her. "I'm sorry," he said, and walked past her into the living room without removing his coat or boots.

Alice followed him. "Henry, are you all right?"

"No, Mom. Everything's a mess." He sat down on the chesterfield, his head bent low.

Tom doused his half-smoked cigarette in the ashtray on the side table. "Son," he said, "what's the matter?"

Henry looked from his mother to his father, then back to a blank spot on the wall. "It's gone," he whispered. "I'm really sorry. You didn't even know."

Alice and Tom exchanged a look, waiting for an explanation. When none came, Alice sat next to her son. "Know what?" She tugged on his arm. "What's gone?"

Henry continued to stare ahead, his eyes glazed over. "Maybe it's my fault."

Tom leaned toward his son, trying to make eye contact. "We don't understand what you're talking about."

Henry's gaze drifted to his father. "I should've told you, but I couldn't."

"Please," Tom said. "You're not making any sense."

"I knew you'd come 'round."

"Come around to what?"

"Me being a doctor."

"Yes?"

"But . . . I decided against it. You couldn't understand why."

"Yes," Mike said. "It was quite a shock."

"I couldn't tell you before because . . ." He paused as if unsure of what to say next. " . . . because Mary asked me not to." Henry's right heel tapped the floor. "She is pregnant, having our baby. I asked her to marry me, but she refused."

Tom and Alice gaped at each other.

Mike spoke up. “I take it she doesn’t want to ruin your chance to be a doctor.”

Henry nodded. “Every time I tried to talk to her she turned me away.”

“Love,” Alice said softly. “It’s gone, you said.”

“The—”

The front door smacked against the wall and Mary burst into the house. “Henry, I must talk to you right away.” Her cheeks burned scarlet. “You and me, alone.” She looked at Tom and Alice. “It’s very important.” Her chest heaved.

Tom grabbed his crutches. “We’ll be in the kitchen. Come on, Alice.” Mike followed them from the room.

“Mary,” Henry said as soon as the others had left. “What are you doing here?” He led her to the chesterfield. “Sit down. You shouldn’t be out of bed in your condition.”

“I still can’t believe I did it.” The groove between Mary’s brows deepened. “It was mean and cruel. You’ll never be able to forgive me.”

“It’s not your fault you lost the baby. Maybe if I hadn’t hounded you all . . .” Henry left the sentence unfinished.

Mary started to rock. “You can’t blame yourself. Oh, Henry, I’ve made such a mess of everything.”

Henry stroked her cheek. “No you haven’t.”

“I lied about the baby.”

“What? I . . .” Henry shook his head. “Lied about the baby? It . . . doesn’t make any sense.” He ran a hand through his hair.

“I’m so sorry.”

“You refused to marry me. Why pretend you were pregnant?”

Mary burst into tears. "You don't understand. I was pregnant."

"Then what are you trying to say?"

Mary pulled a tissue from her pocket and wiped her nose. "I'm still pregnant. I didn't miscarry."

"You lied about the miscarriage," Henry whispered, his bottom lip quivering.

"I was confused, desperate."

Henry stood up, staring at Mary as if she were a stranger. "What kind of game are you playing?"

"It was wrong of me. I realize that now."

"Why did you do it?" Henry barked.

"I couldn't bear to marry a man who only wanted to give his child a name."

Henry's eyes narrowed. "I don't know who you are anymore."

Mary's fingernails dug into the palms of her hands, puncturing the flesh. "I deserve your anger. But I'd rather be alone than be hurt the way my mother was."

"The lie was your way of getting rid of me," Henry snapped. "To hell with our baby."

"No. It was a test to see if you really wanted me for me."

Henry laughed, a guttural, unpleasant sound. "A test. How could you do that?"

"I felt shoved aside like a used dishrag when you applied for medical school. Then the fire happened and all those people died." Mary sobbed. "When I found your grandmother dead, it hurt so bad. Then the roof caved in on both of us." Her voice shook. "My life's been turned upside down and I can't think straight."

"A lot of people's lives have been turned upside down," Henry said, his voice cold. He turned to leave.

"Henry, don't go. I realize now that you really do love me." She swallowed to ease the lump growing in her throat. "Has my deceit put an end to that?"

Henry looked back at Mary's puffy red eyes, the tear-stained cheeks, and the blonde hair in disarray. He went into the hall without uttering a single word.

Tom and Mike sat at the table smoking. Four butts and smouldering ashes filled an ashtray. Alice wiped down the countertops for the fifth time, scrubbing away at invisible stains. "Is everything all right?" she said when Henry stopped just inside the door, standing as motionless as an ice sculpture.

Tom tried to stand up without his crutches and plopped back into the chair. "You look winded, like you've been kicked in the guts."

"Can you all come back to the living room?" Henry waited for them to follow him.

Tom's crutches thumped down the long hallway, loud in the awkward quietness.

Mary wrung her hands as the silent group seated themselves.

Alice sat on the arm of her husband's chair. "Goodness," she said, "there's enough tension in this room to sink a steamship. It must be awful bad news."

"Now, love," Tom said in a calm voice. "Don't look for trouble. Let's hear Henry out."

Henry moved to the chesterfield and stood over Mary. She looked up at him, her eyes pleading. He sat down. "It's not bad news, Mom. At least I hope you won't think so." Henry took Mary's hand and held it to his chest. "We're going to have a baby."

There was a silent pause, broken by Tom. "And?"

"He wants to get married," Mary said.

Alice inhaled deeply. "How long have you known about the baby?"

"The day before the fire, Mrs. Gibbs. Henry found out after I came home from the hospital."

Henry looked at both his parents. "You're some calm about this. Why aren't you shocked, surprised?"

"Love," Alice said. "You don't reach our age with your head stuck in a paper bag."

"That's the truth of it," Tom said. "The sudden decision to drop medical school had to be prompted by an awful big event. The possibility of a baby did cross our minds."

"Why didn't you confront me?"

"Because you're not a boy anymore."

Mary covered her face with her hands. "I've made a mess of everything."

Alice put her arms around the young woman. "Don't look so ashamed. It's not the end of the world."

"Dr. Kennedy said the same thing. Oh, Mrs. Gibbs, I've done an unforgivable thing."

"Nonsense, child. You didn't make the baby on your own."

"That's not what I mean." Mary glanced at Henry. "I—"

"Mary won't marry me," Henry said quickly. "She doesn't want to hold me back from becoming a doctor."

Tom lit a cigarette. "I have only one question for you, Henry. If Mary doesn't become your wife, will you go to medical school?"

Alice gasped. "Tom, what kind of a question is that, especially in front of Mary?"

"Please answer the question, Henry."

"I won't run away from my child for any reason."

"You heard him, Mary," Tom said. "There's no reason to put my son off any longer."

Mike sat with his elbows resting on the arms of the chair. "If I may be permitted to make an observation." All eyes turned to him. "Why does it have to be one way or the other? Can't we all work together to find a solution that will get both these young people what they want?"

HENRY WALKED MARY HOME. "Why didn't you tell your parents about my horrible lie?" she asked.

"To what end? I can only imagine how hard it was on your family when your father ran off."

Mary stopped and faced Henry. "I would never keep our baby from you or your parents, no matter what you decided about us."

"For the last time, Mary, please hear what I've been trying to tell you from the beginning. I want to give our baby a respectable start in life for two reasons."

"Which are?"

"The baby deserves both parents."

"That's one reason. What's the other?"

"I love you."

"BREAKFAST WAS WONDERFUL AS USUAL, Mrs. Simms," Mike said, patting his stomach. "I've gained weight since I've been here."

"A few extra pounds never hurt anyone," the housekeeper said. She looked down at her own voluminous waistline. "I can outwork any skinny young lass."

"I don't doubt it in the least."

"Besides," Mrs. Simms added, "you need some fat to keep warm in this cold weather."

Dr. Kennedy pushed his eggs and bacon around the plate.

Mrs. Simms folded her arms. "What's gotten into you, Doctor? Any other time I'd have a second helping served by now."

"I'm not hungry. Maybe a nice hot cup of tea will do the trick."

"Right away," Mrs. Simms said, taking away the empty teapot.

"Frankie," Mike said, "you've been sullen and withdrawn since yesterday. Does it have anything to do with the release of the Emerson report on the fire?"

"Afraid so. Emerson found Isaac Hull directly responsible for the fire because he was careless over the stove." Dr. Kennedy threw his napkin over his cold breakfast. "Not enough staff and lack of a fire escape contributed to the many deaths which were all Isaac's responsibility."

"How's the man holding up?"

"I dropped by his house after the report came out. His wife laid into me about how unfairly her husband has been judged. She accused me of standing on the sidelines instead of defending him."

"It's understandable she's upset, but you could only tell the truth."

"You're right, of course, yet . . ."

"Yet nothing."

"I was the Home's doctor and medical adviser. Perhaps I should share some of the blame."

"Don't be absurd, Frankie."

"I suggested to Isaac that he needed to hire more nurses. But I didn't press the issue."

"According to what Henry told me about both of the Hulls,

it wouldn't have made one inkling of a difference if you had sung it from the rooftop."

"City Hall and the Health and Welfare Department were equally criticized for not enforcing the improvements which were needed." Dr. Kennedy shoved his plate aside like it was an annoyance. "No one in a position of power cared enough about the sick and old to make sure they were safe." He looked at Mike. "What does that say about us as a society?"

"Hopefully it'll wake the government up to the realization that changes must be implemented to protect those unable to care for themselves."

"Why does it always take a disaster?"

"We won't allow ourselves to envision the worst, especially if money is involved. Do you know if criminal charges will be laid against Mr. Hull?"

"Afraid not," Dr. Kennedy said. "Which isn't going to sit real well with anyone."

Mike couldn't hide his surprise. "How did he accomplish that feat?"

"Manslaughter charges are only brought against a person if they neglect safety with the knowledge that human life is at risk. Sir Emerson believes that Isaac Hull was negligent, yet didn't really consider the full implications entailed by that neglect."

"I guess Emerson has to go by the letter of the law," Mike said. "Still, it must be hard for family and friends of the deceased to accept."

Dr. Kennedy nodded. "Civil suits can be brought against him. We'll have to wait and see if anyone does."

"Do you think Alice will bring one?"

"It's not in her nature. As far as she's concerned, Dot's gone.

Dragging the Hulls through court for what could turn out to be years won't be worth whatever compensation she might win."

Mrs. Simms laid a fresh pot of tea on the table. "Dr. Gibbs." She tutted. "Your missus will be at the airport, luggage in hand, thinking you've forgotten about her."

Mike rose from the table. "Thank you for the reminder, Mrs. Simms."

"A bit of good luck," Dr. Kennedy said, the twinkle back in his eyes. "Lilah's right on time for the wedding."

Chapter 21

DOUGIE, DRESSED IN A BORROWED suit, walked Mary down the aisle. Flora sat with Alice and Tom in the first pew. "Dougie looks some grown up," Flora said, a handkerchief to her eyes. "He looks more like his father every day." She raised her eyes to the crucifix above the altar. "Thank the Lord that's where the resemblance ends."

Father Whitten smiled at the boy. "Who gives this woman in matrimony?"

Dougie stood tall. "Me and Mom do." Mary kissed his cheek and handed her white roses to Jean Baker.

"You look beautiful," Henry said as Mary stood next to him.

The ceremony began with Alice and Flora wiping their eyes often, stopping only when they reached the reception for family and a few close friends. The meal of stuffed chicken was a big hit with everyone.

"That's a lovely pale green suit your daughter is wearing," Lilah Gibbs said as Mary and Henry danced together for the first time as man and wife. "It's very flattering. She could be featured in a fashion magazine."

"Mary is a picture to behold," Flora said, her eyes watering.

"Ah, Mom," Dougie said. "Don't start bawling again."

Fred Russell had left his bakery job an hour early to attend the wedding. He held his head up proudly. "They sure do make a handsome couple."

Lilah Gibbs smiled. "They certainly do."

Fred unbuttoned his jacket, which was made a little more snug from the two plates of dinner he devoured before anyone had finished the first. "Henry will make a fine doctor one day. Always said the boy was destined for good things."

"Tell me, Fred." He had earlier insisted Lilah call him by his Christian name. "Have you any children?"

Fred beamed. "Indeed I do," he said, and held up seven fingers.

"What a large family."

"Not in these parts, it ain't. We had one every year. The oldest is twenty-six on down to twenty. Four boys, three girls. All married and living in town." He made a face. "Still waiting on grandchildren."

"Your wife couldn't make the wedding?"

"Her mother's a mite under the weather. My missus is gone around the bay to look after her."

Tom leaned into Mike. "You'd better rescue Lilah," he whispered. "Fred will talk her ear off."

Mike cocked his head to the side. "She's loving every second."

The music ended. Henry and Mary walked to the table, the groom's arm around his bride's waist. "That's enough dancing for one night," he said, pulling out a chair for Mary.

Lilah stood up. "Both of you come with me," she said. "I want a private word."

Tom gazed at Mike. "What's that all about?" he said,

watching his son and new daughter-in-law follow Lilah across the dance floor.

Mike smiled as if he had learned a secret no one else knew. "My dear wife is always up to something."

Lilah headed toward the female washroom.

"I can't go in there, " Henry said, coming to an abrupt halt at the door.

"Who's going to stop you?" Lilah said, herding him and Mary inside.

Henry's eyes darted around the room. "Someone might come in."

"That's easy enough to remedy," Lilah said, and locked the door. "Now we won't be disturbed."

"But . . ." Henry's voice trailed away when Mary giggled.

Lilah took in the newlyweds with one glance. "Mike told me all about your dilemma."

Mary blushed all the way down to her neck.

"My girl," Lilah said. "You've nothing to be ashamed of. When Mike and I were married I was three months in the family way. In the family way," she repeated. "I do love that expression."

"Mrs. Gibbs," Henry said.

"Call me Aunt Lilah."

"Aunt Lilah, I don't feel at home in here. What is it you want to discuss with us?"

"A baby is a precious gift, not something that hinders what you want from life."

Henry took Mary's hand in his. "The difference between our situation and yours is that your uncle Mike was a practising doctor and making good money at the time."

"Let's get down to it," Lilah continued. "We're all family. Will you allow Mike and me to help?"

"That's generous of you," Henry said. "But I won't take any handouts."

Mary smiled up at Henry. "My husband is a proud man."

The door handle rattled. Henry jumped. "A woman's trying to get in."

"All full," Lilah called, and turned back to Henry and Mary. "You misunderstand. I'm offering both of you a way to earn your own money. Mary, your mother showed me the most exquisite quilt I've ever seen. One that you made."

"Anyone can make quilts."

"Not in Toronto, my dear. I doubt you'd be able to keep up with the orders." Lilah winked. "And I'm acquainted with the right circle of money people. Henry," she carried on, to prevent either one from voicing an objection, "you planned on working part-time anyway."

"On my own, renting a small room, it would work." He pulled Mary closer. "A house is another issue altogether."

"You could stay with us."

"No," Mary said. "That would be too much of an intrusion."

"I agree," Henry said.

"You young people," Lilah sighed. "Always reaching the wrong conclusion without waiting for all the information. We have a furnished apartment over the garage. Our oldest son and his wife lived there until they could afford to buy a house. You can have it rent-free, as they did." She put up a hand to stall an objection. "If that's unsuitable, you and my husband can come to a suitable payment."

"You hardly know us," Mary said.

"In all the time I've been with my husband, he's never been this happy or at peace. Please don't disappoint him."

Henry studied his new aunt. "Tell me," he said. "How come Uncle Mike didn't talk to us himself?"

"It's like this, love." Lilah smiled. "I really do love your Newfoundland expressions. This is my way of proving that I'm one hundred per cent behind the plan." She unlocked the door. "Actually," she added, "I thought up the brilliant idea."

"WELL?" MIKE SAID WHEN LILAH rejoined him at the table.

She turned to the young couple on the floor, who were doing a jig to "All Around the Circle." Fred and Flora danced next to them, kicking up their heels with the energy of youngsters.

Mike put a hand on her chin and turned her face to him. "Lilah, what happened?"

"Sweetheart, when have I ever not gotten my way?"

"Thank you," Mike said, and kissed her cheek. "By the way, did I ever tell you why I chose you to be my wife?"

Lilah raised her eyebrows in mock surprise. "Because I won you over, of course."

"It's because you reminded me of a Newfoundlander."

"Did you tell Tom and Alice about the plan yet?"

"He did," Tom said, coming to the table with whiskies for him and Mike. He looked out at the dance floor and sighed. "My son the doctor." He smiled at Alice. "Has a nice ring to it, don't you think?"

Alice laughed out loud.

Tom stared at her. "What's so funny?"

She hugged him. "Nothing at all, Henry, love. Nothing at all.

Acknowledgements

Thanks once again to Paul Butler for his expertise and guidance. A special thanks to my mother for her first-hand knowledge of the fire and the devastating effect on the community. And thank you to Garry Cranford and Jerry Cranford for giving me the opportunity to share this story.

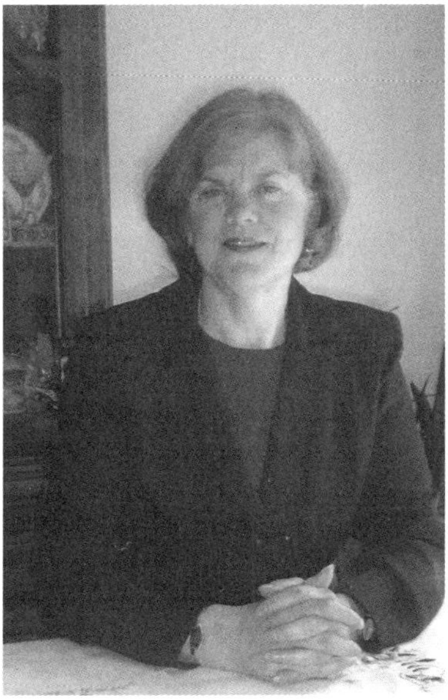

LINDA ABBOTT was born in St. John's, the eighth in a family of ten children. She is a graduate of Memorial University, with a Bachelor of Arts and Education. She holds a Certificate in French from Laval University, Quebec City, and attended the Frecker Institute in St. Pierre. She is a retired French Immersion teacher, having spent most of her career at Holy Trinity Elementary School in Torbay. *The Hull Home Fire* is her second novel. Her first novel was the critically acclaimed bestseller *The Loss of the Marion*. She resides in St. John's.

MIX
Paper from
responsible sources
FSC® C103567
FSC
www.fsc.org